‘Part memoir, part advice, all inspiration’

CANCER UNHINGED

Tony Dehn and Sally Dehn

Published by Dehn Family Publishing

Paperback edition - ISBN: 978-0-6488838-0-7

Kindle edition - ISBN: 978-0-6488838-1-4

ePub edition - ISBN: 978-0-6488838-2-1

DISCLAIMER

The information, strategies, concepts, techniques, and suggestions in this book are of a general nature only, and do not constitute, and are not intended as a substitute for, professional or individual advice in any way. You should consult with the appropriate qualified professionals (including psychologists, psychiatrists, counsellors, medical practitioners and other healthcare providers, insurance advisers, financial advisers, and legal advisers) and seek your own independent professional advice relating to your particular circumstances and needs.

Although the author and the publisher have made every effort to ensure that the contents of this book were accurate at press time, the author and the publisher do not represent or warrant their accuracy. The author and the publisher are not responsible for any disruption, loss or damage (including indirect or consequential damages) suffered by any party as a result of, or in relation to, the use of this book. To the extent permitted by law, the author and the publisher exclude any liability (including liability for negligence or other default) to any party for any disruption, loss or damage (including indirect or consequential damages) arising from or in relation to the use of this book.

DEDICATION

For every person dealing with a terminal diagnosis – we hope it helps.

CONTENTS

FOREWORD

It is an honour to be invited to write a foreword for Cancer Unhinged.

I am familiar throughout its subjects and contents; I feel myself part of its fabric and matrix, and it strikes close to home.

Anthony Ernest Dehn (Tony) is my brother-in-law; Sally my sister.

I have known them as individuals and as a formidable, inseparable team forever. We have lived and grown together, journeyed on many enquiries and quests together; our families grew up together. I have observed from near and far how their bond weaves their work, as a partnership and as individuals. They are of similar mind, and share amazing support for each other, both demonstrated and tacit.

Foreword is an apt term, as a homonym, when considering their approach to the bombshell that landed when Tony had only just turned 54. Immediately, while the dust was yet contemplating its fall on an uncertain future, there were investigations into what exactly was wrong, how it was to be righted and, at each stage, when the next step would be taken. There were practical limitations and implications, adjustments to be made to ways of living, to dreams and expectations. Daily Life demanded to continue even while it was turned on its head; the threat of despair lurked at every turn.

Their tale catalogues actions and reactions, emotions, philosophies, and psychologies... and practical measures, important to share with a person facing cancer or for those supporting someone battling cancer. That's a given. What wins through, however, is the display of human spirit which underlies this gift, this legacy. There is not a shred of 'give-up' anywhere in these pages: there is anger, confusion, frustration, resolution, absolution, but at no point is there submission.

The value in illustrating the stark realities of facing premature death and sharing a unique outlook without any emphasis or pretence of bravery, is to display that the greatest weapon available against this desperation is attitude – not stated, but demonstrated.

This communicates beyond the victims of cancer – there is a strong case, for anyone who realises they may one day die, to read this book.

INTRODUCTION

This book is a manual for those who've been told they are going to die. And a handbook for those who walk alongside. It comprises the thoughts and insights of cancer experiencer Tony Dehn and his wife Sally, written from the horse's back, so to speak. Throughout the book, you'll find sections by each of them, with their name at the start of each, so you know whose 'voice' you are reading. Some of what you'll read will be their description of the journey, and some, particularly from Tony, is the thoughts that were written down then, as everything happened.

If you've been given a use-by date, this book can help you free yourself from the anguish of the diagnosis of a premature death.

This book is for....

- People with use-by dates.
- Loved ones of people with use-by dates
- For healthy men.

This book was written...

- To bring into one place a collection of thoughts on topics and spaces that I experienced on my journey into the realm of uncertainty and grief after being told I would be dead sometime soon.
- For people who have been dealt the news that they are going to die soon.
- To provide an easy-to-comprehend layman's description of what cancer is and what it is not.
- To lighten the mental/ psychological load of people who have been told they have a use-by date.

- To provide a perspective for people who don't have a use-by date, to allow them access to what is typically going on for the person who has been given a use-by date.
- To provide a (mental) get-out-of-jail-free card which will bring freedom from the psychological imprisonment of 'you're gonna be getting dead soon'.
- To free people from the societal pressure to declare 'depression'.
- To have people realise it's ok to smile in the face of death.
- To provide you steps towards freeing yourself from the despair of death.
- To have you 'get' that you're NOT just basically human trash because you have cancer.
- To provide a *real, direct,* and *authentic* straight talk from someone who's riding the horse.

My wish is for you to read this book and then gift or share a copy with someone you know who's dealing with cancer. If you don't know anyone with cancer, give it to any healthy man, in the hopes that he will hear the advice within its pages, and go get his prostate checked, before it is too late.

In this book I try to address the 'unanswerable' questions people have about a diagnosis of terminal cancer, including addressing the following concerns for yourself or your loved ones.

- How will it affect my family?
- How will I cope with the treatment?
- How will I cope with losing a body part?
- Am I going to die?
- What is death?
- How do I tell people I've got cancer?
- What kind of financial support is available?
- How do I handle being told I'm going to die?
- How do I know if what they're telling me is the truth?
- What do I do with the rest of my life while I'm waiting for this thing to take me out?
- How do I deal with people's well-meaning intentions and non-thinking reactions when I tell them I have terminal cancer?
- The life lessons that come into play the day of diagnosis.

In reading this book and because of it, if you have cancer, a use-by date, or love someone with a use-by date, I expect you to let go of the riverbank of life, to jump into the river and roll and swim and play along with me as we delve into spaces and places unknown to you or I...

There are ways of making you do this... jump in before you get pushed...

Why?

Because if you jump you take the power to control how you deal with what the river of life brings you... and if you wait to be pushed you and your power get separated.

And you'll struggle and won't know why you're struggling...

Be loud, proud and in love with life....

Tony Dehn

A Note from Sally Dehn

When I started looking for support after my husband was diagnosed with prostate cancer, I found it very limited. I joined an online forum, seeking company and solace in this lonely world of being my husband's carer, to find that it was like plucking hairs out of a chicken

Yes, family and friends offered their support, however a lot of them couldn't deal with it at all and we were the ones who were holding them up a majority of the time.

Just maybe sharing our story will make a difference to yours.

This is not aimed to be a sad and depressing account of our journey with cancer, it is aimed to provide tools and assistance for those who may be going through a similar situation by unhinging the power we sometimes give the C word.

If you are interested in learning a bit about our lives, before cancer entered the scene, see the 'About the Author' section at the back of this book. Now, strap in for the story of our roller-coaster ride...

CHAPTER 1 - SOME FACTS...

If you're over 40 and you're male, you need to know...

Prostate cancer takes out (KILLS) 9 men every day in Australia.

And the prognosis is the same tomorrow and... we don't have a cure.

Prostate Cancer doesn't care

- How healthy you are...
- What race or colour you are...
- Or what you eat for dinner...

If you're male and you're over 40... You may be next!

It kills indiscriminately... if you get it, and it doesn't kill you directly, it will directly contribute to you killing yourself.

- The suicide rate of men with cancer is four times the national average.
- Each year in Australia, over 3,000 men are killed by prostate cancer.
- Around 20,000 men are diagnosed in Australia every year with prostate cancer.
- Rural men are 20% more likely to get cancer than city people
- 1 in 1000 men aged 40+ will get prostate cancer
- 12 out of every 1,000 men over the age of 50 will get prostate cancer
- 45 out of every 1000 men over 60 will get prostate cancer

In Australia, prostate cancer kills more men than breast cancer kills women. This insidious disease is sneaky... and deadly... it will get you...

If you don't get it first.

Prostate cancer is often seen as an 'old man's disease', especially by men themselves. But cancer is NOT just an old man's disease, it is a REAL man's disease, a 'he-man's' disease, and a bloke's disease. It can happen to ANY man, at ANY age!

The 'he-man' cultural phenomenon, that blokey, men's-club type attitude prevalent in Western culture, contributes heavily to the late diagnosis of prostate cancer.

Death rates can be lowered if real men bravely girl-up' against this insidious, sneaky disease.

If you are a man and you'd like the best chance of avoiding it, and surviving it if it gets you... then this book is for you, too.

CHAPTER 2 - FACT OR FICTION

Sally

Symptoms: Happy 54th Birthday

Looking back to when we first learned about Tony's cancer seems a lifetime ago. I have a vivid memory of Tony going to the GP as he was having difficulty urinating, experiencing pain in the lower back, which he had been to the chiropractor about many times, with the chiropractor telling him he didn't think the pain was coming from his back but was actually referred pain.

PSA tests

The GP asked a series of questions and did a blood test for PSA (Prostate-Specific Antigen) level as well as a physical prostate check. The initial response from the GP was to refer Tony straight to a urologist - he said that the prostrate was very hard. To tell you the truth, I had heard of the prostate, but had no idea what its functions were.

Tony was fortunate to get in to see the specialist quite quickly. Sitting in the full waiting room, I thought 'wow, this is a really busy practice', once again not having any idea of what I was just about to learn.

The specialist explained that Tony's PSA level was at 540, and a normal level was... 4. He also said that with a reading as high as that, it was likely that the cancer had spread to other parts of the body, which meant that the cancer couldn't be taken out of the prostate (that is: inoperable). He then booked Tony in for a procedure which would give him an indication of the grading of the cancer.

We were due to go on a cruise in 4 days' time.

The first test

The specialist advised us to go on our cruise and enjoy ourselves (as if we could after this news) and book into the procedure for when we return. We did go on the cruise, attempting to enjoy ourselves, as we actually at this stage knew what we were facing.

On return, Tony had the procedure, showing that the cancer had spread into his lymph glands and was spreading into his bladder and kidneys.

The prognosis without treatment: a life expectancy of less than a year, with female hormone treatment 2-3 years.

So now we had the full picture, sitting in the specialist's rooms, with the specialist apologising to Tony when he delivered the news.

I was in shock.

I know that the tears sprang to my eyes, and thoughts of 'what are we going to do? How are we going to tell the kids? It is going to be alright, isn't it???'

My mind was consumed with unanswered questions. I found myself holding it together for the kids and Tony, but crying myself to sleep on a daily basis with thoughts of how we were going to get through this.

Tony

My name is Tony Dehn. I am 54 years young (note, this section was written in 2013). I have been married 27 years, and have 3 teenagers. I have been self-employed for 30+ years. I live on the Gold Coast in Queensland, Australia.

In 2008 I had a prostate check-up and was given the all clear. In January 2013 I was diagnosed with TERMINAL AGGRESSIVE PROSTATE CANCER.

According to my specialist, without treatment I will most probably be dead inside twelve months. The cancer has spread beyond the prostate to the lymph nodes and is growing up to the bladder and kidneys. It has not yet gone to the bone.

According to the specialist there is only one proven treatment that can slow this cancer down and that is to take away its food source, which is testosterone.

And the way to kill off the testosterone is with female hormones.

But he said if I take this current treatment, which I am still doing as I write, I will still most probably be pushing up daisies inside three years.

Our Government promotes a 'get tested every two years' campaign. I didn't do that and I'm sure there are many men who are avoiding getting a test because of some irrational 'He-Man' issues about getting an anal examination or 'showing the doc ya bits'.

My hope is to get out a message out to men over the age of fifty to get a prostate check-up.

Becoming a Date Star

In the past I was a 'He-Man' - embarrassed to show my bits to the doctor. I was embarrassed to bare my arse. I thought it was gay - may be for some, but not for me!

Then I saw the blood test report of 540... 540 when it should have been 4.

Tony's Thoughts

Now, three fingers later, my ring's still intact, but my manhood isn't...

I'm a Date Star...

Hot flushes... crying fits... female tits...

It's only a blood test... save yourself while you still can, man...

It wasn't gonna get me but it did...

Wasn't something to be worried about, but it was...

It still got me...

Even through my 'He-Man' shield...

Girl up, boys... unless you're up for eating chocky cake on the couch with me...

But before you risk a visit... Take it from this 'He-Girl'...

It's not all it's cracked up to be over here in the sisterhood.

It looks good from Mansville... but it sucks big time... matter of fact, hot flushes suck....

'No more sex please, I've got a headache' is now my story...

Sorry for being crude and gory, but that's my story...

So, if you like being man... Man up to the doc, show him ya cock,

Risk the finger to check ya prostate... who knows, you may be lucky and get a green light so you can stay stuck in the world of men...

Sorry girls, hope you forgive me for the unladylike language... but I thought the boys needed to know what it's like over here... In your land of no beer.

Please help kill a tree in honour of me...

Print this out and give it to your man to ponder over the next time he opens a beer (or ignores his medical responsibilities....)

...More wine girls?

CHAPTER 3 – TIME SUCKERS

Sally

Doctor Who?

We went to work shortly after the diagnosis understanding that whoever we may be referred to might be a bit of a lottery, as our knowledge (like many others who find themselves in this situation) was very limited; my knowledge of cancer from dealing with mum was that there were many cancer specialists.

As Tony's cancer was in the prostate, we were first referred to a urologist, a physician who has a specialised knowledge in male reproductive organs.

Once he diagnosed us we were then referred to a medical oncologist in Brisbane, so off we went to meet the oncologist for the first time. The waiting room was packed once again, similar to a cattle yard.

I had a sense of overwhelm, not knowing what to expect, knowing that I had zilch knowledge of what we were dealing with, though I had googled about the doctor who we had been referred to, so I did know that he travels the world seeking the latest treatments and has headed up leading trials, so I was comforted to know that this guy knew his stuff...

We were greeted by Dr Mainwaring and his personal assistant. A picture of Tony's MRI results showing where the cancer had spread to was on a large screen.

My memory of what was discussed is a blur. Tony asked a lot of questions as he had a lot more knowledge about what was happening than I did.

The doctor made it very clear that at this stage there is no cure for prostate cancer.

What they did know was that there were several treatments available to Tony to help shrink the cancer, including female hormone therapy called 'androgen deprivation therapy' (ADT), the goal being to reduce levels of male hormones called androgens, or to stop them from affecting prostate cancer cells. In prostate cancer the main androgens are testosterone and dihydrotestosterone (DHT). Now, if you are anything like me trying to understand this information, you need a university degree. A good idea is to record the conversations on your brief visits or take notes.

CHAPTER 4 – FAMILY MATTERS

Sally

Telling the family

The kids dealt with the news in a very matter-of-fact way.

Our eldest took on the responsibility role, and then tended to shut himself away. Our middle child was convinced that her dad was going to die very soon.

I think this came as a result of the visual evidence of Tony not looking very well; he actually looked sick at this point. Our youngest didn't want to talk about it and made jokes where he could.

Then there's family. Tony made it very clear that he was not up for feeling sorry for himself. He also was clear on not wanting to hear the latest unproven cure; it was ok for those who wanted to go down that road but it wasn't going to be for Tony.

Tony is from a large family of eight. He is the eldest of six siblings, always the 'big' brother, though you wouldn't call his relationship with his siblings close. A couple of years ago Tony received a call from one of his younger brothers, with the news that he had prostate cancer with a PSA of 7 and that he was going to get it taken out. I suppose that was our first introduction to prostate cancer. Tony read up on it a lot, gaining an understanding about it which assisted connecting him with his brother. Other than that Tony had very limited conversations with his siblings.

So, facing sharing this news to his family certainly altered the relationships with his siblings. I remember going to a Christmas function when we returned from our holiday, still waiting for final results.

Tony appeared sick, had lost weight, and looked very drawn. He told his family what he knew; in denial he also played down the future we might be or might not be looking into.

I know I was still in shock myself and really didn't want to hold conversations, being asked questions to which I didn't have the answer. Yes, I was certainly in denial too.

Well-meaning thoughts from friends and family

My family has a history of cancer. We had lost my mother to leukaemia six years earlier. Tony's diagnosis brought up a lot of memories not just for me but for the rest of the siblings.

It is hard to keep to the facts when you are telling people of your own situation, as whoever you are talking to always knows someone who has either got, had or passed away from cancer.

The normal flow of conversation and the want of others to contribute sometimes detracts from the communication of simple facts and emotions.

Tony

How does one not worry about what people might say or think about you?

Simple, but not easy.

Getting to there requires getting that there is nowhere to get to...

Releasing worries over what people may or may not say about you requires unlearning and acknowledgement of our human hardwiring.

First you acknowledge that most people, if not all, rarely think. Ninety nine percent of the time we are having thoughts, but thoughts are not necessarily thinking. Thinking is done when one has a challenge or problem that calls for a solution.

If you're not trying to solve a real problem (real means 'will make a difference in someone else's life') then you are merely thought-ing, not thinking!

And your thought-ing about whether or not people care or don't care about what you have to say or not say, are thoughts...and any conclusions drawn from thought-ing is more thought-ing.

These thoughts are not the truth, but for some strange survival reasoning they occur to us as truth.

Those thoughts are not facts. Those thoughts are, however, normal machinations of the human brain's hard-wired need to predict the future. And it does that by having thoughts about thoughts.

One of these thought traps or loops is used by our brains to attempt to predict whether one is liked or not liked...its job is to seek out and it gives us ways to survive and contribute value in our tribes or communities.

Next, one must get that acknowledgment is the currency of the brain. For from acknowledgement, our brains draw survival juice. Our brains think acknowledgement gives us a value in our tribes, which it interprets as a contribution to our ongoing survival on the planet and in our groups.

Acknowledgment is however a bankrupt currency that is devoid of the satisfaction that it so willingly promises. That's why the chase is always more fun than the result.

And the final part is understanding that neither you or I or anyone has any interest in anyone or anything except for themselves.

For the brain knows that without us there is no them...and we twist that into another false truth, called 'there is a meaning to my existence and to my life...'

And there you have it. When you give up the idea you once clung to, that your life has a 'meaning', and that it doesn't mean anything that your life has no meaning, then and only then, the worries about whether people like you or not dissipate into the nothingness from whence they came.

CHAPTER 5 – CANCER DOESN'T CARE

Tony

3-month update

In January 2013, three months ago, I was confirmed as having aggressive prostate cancer that had left the prostate and travelled to the lymph glands and was growing into my bladder and kidneys.

The prognosis was that without treatment life expectancy was less than 1 year; with female hormone treatment I could possibly expect 2-3 years.

I chose the hormone ride.

Results after treatment confirmed that the hormone ride has extended my life ride to the 2-3-year option. Lucky me...

Tests, Scans, MRI

The PSA level was 540; it's now 0.97 which confirms that the hormone treatment has shut down the testosterone production. I am now officially a Toni. Hot flushes, mood swings, no sex drive...

Scans and X-rays reveal shrinkage of the prostate and its growths and lymph node tumours by 60%. However, there is persistent thickening of the bladder wall on the right-hand side (this is possibly another tumour growth, yet to be confirmed).

There are no new lesions.

End of report.

Now to what you can do to help and to all who responded to my initial announcement in January...

'I'm with you, Toni...'

Thanks for your thoughts and good wishes...

Now it's time to empower me and support me and prove you're with me. To prove you're with me, please help me hit my target:

1000 X 50+ aged men being tested and being given a green light...

To support me, what would really make a difference is that when you have twisted a man's arm to go get a test... (Please understand - they need twisting because most He-Men won't go) ...that you join the green light man to my 1000 green lights stories.

To be updated you can visit this free-range human on Facebook. Every time I see a new green light story I get empowered to fight on. If you've already been tested as a result of my sharing please go there now and tell me your story.

Again I thank you for your support and well wishes,

Toni...

Rant time

Cancer doesn't care about memories, who you're friends with, how many friends you have, how peaceful or angry you are or are not; who you love, or if you even love. It doesn't care if you have faith, hope and belief in an almighty.

Cancer doesn't care for our human rules... cancer is us. Cancer is our own cell survival mechanism doing what the inventor of humans designed it to do. Cancer is cells continuing to divide as they are genetically programmed to do.

There is nothing wrong with cancer or with having cancer.

There is nothing wrong with me because cancer is in existence in my body. In fact, having cancer in my body makes me *present* to how human I am. It gives understanding of what it is to be human as it focuses the mind on what's most important for the continuance of my human existence.

... When I'm dead will I still exist?

These comments are designed to continue my existence in time and space for those who may have an interest in the machinations of the mind of a human who's soon not to be... this is the true life after death.

I have died to faith, to hope, to fantasy, to despair, to hatred, to love, to want, to needing to continue to be alive.

I choose...

I am alive, I am free, I am me; I live, I love, I do, I am, I don't, I am whole, I am an asshole, I am complete, I lack nothing, I am everything and I am nothing.

Life is empty and meaningless and I and my life are empty and meaningless.

And that you make that mean something is empty and meaningless.

To me and to the world:

I am hopeless... I am faithless... I am despair-less.

I am me dealing with getting dead...

What are you dealing with? Hoping to live a great life? Living as others say you should, as you were trained for or duped into? Living in order to get or be a somebody, somewhere, someday.

Be that person today. You are who you say you are. Saying and being who you are carries immense personal power. Do you know you can create a way of being that is unrecognizable to you? Free yourself from the tyranny of hope...

Join me in the world of hopeless human beings.

I now see a world filled with hopeless human beings. A world filled with humans who are aware that they are everything and nothing at the same time...

CHAPTER 6 – STAYING ALIVE

Sally

A close friend of mine said to me, 'You're not the one with the cancer, you cannot know what Tony is going through'.

I remind myself of this daily as it helps me let him go through the emotions, frustrations, and anger in his own way. Of course I care, but I don't try to stop him, as I believe that would be smothering those emotions.

I remember Tony standing at the kitchen sink one day crying, not just crying but crying like someone had died - a grieving cry. At first, I wanted to console him by saying it will be ok. I chose not to; I let him cry. My son's response was one of hugging and supporting. As I said before, there is no right and wrong way of how to live with someone with a terminal disease.

Tony speaks of this event as grieving for the person he was. It also, I believe, allowed him to accept to a certain degree what his life was now. It is very common for cancer patients to shut down their emotions, to stop talking to friends about what they are going through. Often depression and suicidal thoughts take up the space of communication and the sufferer tends to withdraw and become a recluse. Anger is very often present, which usually results in a written rant.

We have made a commitment that when Tony feels like this he speaks out, sharing his thoughts, as that's all they are, just thoughts. He finds that once he does that, the thoughts diminish.

At first, I found this confronting, once again not knowing what to say as I just wanted to fix how he was feeling. I used to start crying in fear he was going to commit suicide.

I then started to just listen without attachment. It might sound a bit cold-hearted, but if I listened and cried, it would be about me. If I listen with the intent of allowing Tony's frustrations and emotions to subside and it not affect me, then I have been there for him.

He does the same for me; we call it the dumping session. If I do get attached by what he is sharing I go and flush the toilet, this way I am flushing the contents of the conversation away and not carrying it with me.

Tony

A psychologist walked around a room while teaching stress management to an audience.

As she raised a glass of water, everyone expected they'd be asked the 'half empty or half full' question. Instead, with a smile on her face, she inquired: 'How heavy is this glass of water?'

Answers called out ranged from 8 oz. to 20 oz.

She replied, 'The absolute weight doesn't matter. It depends on how long I hold it. If I hold it for a minute, it's not a problem. If I hold it for an hour, I'll have an ache in my arm. If I hold it for a day, my arm will feel numb and paralysed. In each case, the weight of the glass doesn't change, but the longer I hold it, the heavier it becomes,' she continued, 'the stresses and worries in life are like that glass of water. Think about them for a while and nothing happens. Think about them a bit longer and they begin to hurt. And if you think about them all day long, you will feel paralysed - incapable of doing anything.'

And you have the sensation and feeling of being stressed.

So what can you do?

As early in the evening as you can, put all your burdens down. Don't carry them through the evening and into the night.

And as you lay down to sleep let them slip into the past. The best place to put the past problems is in the past!

And it takes nothing but losing your stress to leave them there.

Suicidal thoughts

I do expect that this will mess with your head...

So be warned this piece is for humans only...

Non-humans should cease reading now...

The world says you shouldn't have suicidal thoughts, even after you get a terminal diagnosis. But they are already at the party before you arrive. It's part of the journey. Don't resist it – it's not bad to have suicidal thoughts, it's not good. It just IS. Kick it around, play with it, but don't go into the corner and suck your thumb. The thoughts will have you want to go into the corner and feel sorry for yourself. It's not your only option.

Religion and hope and faith say we have to be positive, filled with hope and positivity. Hope and faith, right and wrong, are the root-cause of feelings of inadequacy that rob people of life and of their lives.

Just because you have cancer doesn't mean you are a bad person. It doesn't mean you did anything wrong, it doesn't mean you deserve bad things to happen to you. Cancer lives in a world where it is considered a bad thing. That cancer is bad is our cultural norm. But cancer is a normal function of the body, and it is a natural phenomenon. It didn't happen to you because you thought bad things, because you did bad things, or because you deserve it.

Suicide is an escape from the incessant pain that the false 'religionified' world we live in inflicts on every one of us...but we don't really live in a binary world. There is no 'right' and no 'wrong'. But the cancer and the 'badness' around it is only 'bad' because you label it 'wrong'.

The desire to kill oneself comes from a loss of hope. But hope is not necessarily required to be happy and have a life not unlike the one you had before you were told you have cancer.

Human beings are whole and complete and don't require hope to live fulfilled lives.

Renounce hope...

Renounce all faith...

Renounce the thought that you can get your life wrong.

Renounce the hope of being able to get life right and renounce that life should be going any other way than the way it's going. Its going the way it's going, because that's the way it going. And it was never going to go any other way than the way it has gone.

Renounce that your life has any meaning or value other than to provide food for the worms that will feed on your carcass after your death.

Do this as I have, and you will find freedom from the pain of expectation that the world has been force feeding you since birth.

You will find the real you, and it will be a happy you, who won't require anything from anybody; happiness will be there right in the place it's always been, covered up by the layers of bullshit the world and its ways and its expectations have been heaping on you since birth.

Free yourself from the tyranny of mankind and its societal inventions of what being a human is supposed to look and feel and be like. Renounce all hope of life being any other way than the way it is.

Release yourself from the burden of having to be or to not be a certain way in order to make it with personage or a god that doesn't exist. It will also release you from being a 'you' and the idea that there needs to be a 'you' in order to be able to function in the world...

The truth is, you and I have never had anything to do with how life treats us. Life and the world do what they do without any consideration for their effect on you or I. And it is only our expectation that the world should heed our view that gets us f@?*ed up.

The 'you' that you and I think we are is an invention of our minds. It has no basis in reality and is not required nor has it ever been required in order for us to continue to play on this planet we call home.

Ask yourself the question....

If I was enrolled in every area of my life, what would that look like?

Thank you for your support and well wishes,

Toni ...

Chapter 7 - Don't steal my thunder: A Message to the 4-Me's

Tony

The world is filled with people for whom it's all about them. Six billion of them. I call them the '4-me's'. 4-me's still operate life like there is a tomorrow.

'It's all about me - even your UBD (use-by-date) has somehow got to be made into something about *me* - a story about how I or someone I know did or didn't do something so that I get to feel that I have contributed to the UBD situation.'

Even though, the truth is, all I did was make some noise that sucked away a few minutes of that UBD person's time...

> *NOTE! (Rant interrupt)*
>
> Before I became a UBD I was, and still am, a 4-me; if I wasn't I wouldn't be writing this rant. This rant at its core is all about what I think and what I think *you* should think and do, because I'm over here in the land of UBD.
>
> *Back to Rant...*

4-me's never even consider stopping being a 4-me.

It's impossible: you're hard-wired to do 4-me just as I am. For UBDs understand that 4-me's can't stop it, it's hard-wired. 4-me's, just keep on doing what you're doing, just do more of it.

Here are four simple tips that you as a 4-me can do for a UBD 4-me...

- Refrain from telling a UBD 4-me how you feel about what they're having to deal with.
- Refrain from telling them about someone or something you've heard about.
- Refrain from asking them how they're feeling. UBDs don't need you to refocus them on how they're feeling. They need you to focus them on getting stuff done.
- Refrain from asking them a generalised what can you do for them. Do not ask me that, because if you do, I am going to ask you to pay my mortgage for me. Get specific; invite me to the pub for a beer, invite me to dinner, but don't ask me something I cannot answer right there and then. It is glib, and unanswerable.

Now you know what not to do, here are four tips on what to do:

1. If you want to offer them well-meant advice on what to do to cure their cancer based on your grandmother's special recipe or something you heard on the radio, don't. Get on Google and do six hours research and present them with a one page fact sheet. This will save THEM six hours of their now precious time they have left on this earth. That IS something you can do for them.
2. Find out from their friends/ relatives or the UBD themselves, what things they are trying or wanting to get done and pick one thing. Then request permission from the UBD and do the thing and present the UBD with the result. (Do not tell them anything about how much it took or cost or what was involved.)

   Just show or give them what you did.

   UBDs have no interest in hearing more about how you feel about them, or how much you love them; they already have that for granted. All they have time for is dealing with how they're feeling, and how they can distract themselves from dealing with what they're feeling.

3. Get involved. Don't make a UBD do the research on your hare-brained idea. The UBD probably doesn't have the time, money, education, or the inclination.

   Don't give a UBD positive thinking stories or sayings, or the latest untested cancer 'cure', unless you have the facts to back you up.

Facts are not what someone told you, or what you read or heard or thought sounded good. Did you ponder it, think about it? Did you use *your* time rather than the UBD's time? Did you test it, did you ask for ten opinions? Just beware that even if ten thousand people agree, it still doesn't make a fact.

Facts are like gravity. Every time you throw it up it comes down. Every time the stuff of *fact* is given or taken or thought, it produces a result, every time, and just in case you think 100 is a big ask, 'Works for 80 of the people 80 percent of the time' will do.

BUT not: someone, somewhere, someone said or I heard about Blah, blah, blah!

4. To be of real value to a UBD give them what's been taken away - time.

   To be of use - save or add some time.

   After all, time is the only thing you've got that they now haven't. Spend some of yours doing something for them, something that makes a difference in reality (And I don't mean send flowers or cards). Do something that adds or speeds what gets done in the time they have left with you.

   Refrain from making them spend their remaining time doing things *you* want done. Help them get the things they want done, done with VELOCITY.

Three things UBDs want:

1. Monetary security for their loved ones now and forever.
2. Not having to go to work to keep the family fed.
3. Time to rant and be with friends and family free from the concerns of the other 2 wants.

End of Rant.

Oops... Footer to rant –

PS. If you want to give money, give it to the cancer research foundation at Mater hospital. www.materfoundation.org.au or buy a ball at www.balls4life.com.au. Donate in the hope that a cure can be found so my UBD gets put back where it should be... a bit further away down the track, somewhere closer to where yours is.

That was so.

And now I let it go.

CHAPTER 8 - PARALYSIS BY ANALYSIS

Sally

There are so many opinions available on what is best for the patient, not all of them from medical practitioners, let alone specialists. Would it be easier if we didn't have so many people's opinions on what is best for the patient? Or is it good that we have so many options to choose from? Or do too many ideas and options, all vying for attention, make it paralysing to decide, to choose one or another treatment option?

These are good questions, and we have found this subject very challenging.

From the beginning of Tony's hormone treatment (ADT), there were side-effects that impacted on his life as heavily as simply being given the news that he had a terminal illness. He had to come to terms with having his 'maleness' taken away from him (in order to suspend the life sentence, admittedly). He had to deal with new 'female' emotions (like empathy!) and experience phenomena like hot flushes.

Tony found that largely the medications and treatments he endured left him lethargic. As a very active 'hands-on' person this lack of energy frustrated him and impacted on his ability to work full days, which in turn affected his sense of fulfilment not to mention his ability to provide for his family.

On perhaps a more personal level, he had to deal with his own perceptions and attitudes around sex or rather the lack of male testosterone push for sex, while still having a mental expectation of how much sex he should be having. Not to mention dealing with penal discharge that 'smells like vagina'!

Questioning the experts - have *they* got it right or wrong?

These are the facts and side effects of the treatment we undertook, which of course was the treatment path we had chosen and agreed to. The hormone treatment does damage that is irreparable. Tony can't come back from that. Effectively the medical experts have told us there is only one way to deal with this, that there is only one path of treatment, but it occurred to me often, how do they know? Have they got it right of have we missed something crucial? The anxiety of maybe having missed something was present daily.

Tony

Toni's report:

Latest front-line Man Gland cancer report... two years on.

February 2015.

Blue and yellow smarties are dead. Titties are back in grow mode. Brown smarties still kickin'... and growing...

We took away their food source so the ingenious bastards have set up their own factories to produce their own coconuts....

They now have 0.67 of a gram... was previously 0.47

No reduction recorded as wanted.

Result = Failure...

New defence initiative. Two-pronged defensive strategy:

First - move surveillance team from 13 week to 6 weekly intervals.

Second... at 2 gram levels declare two-pronged trench warfare attack.

1st. Send in the seals to hunt and destroy the hidden coconut factories...

2nd. Dispatch 2nd battalion of troops to fill food supply passages with glue to prevent enemy secondary supply line from feeding the enemy.

Seriously Though...

PSA has risen again despite drugs designed to stop it. The current drug, Zoladex, shuts down testosterone production to starve the cancer but the human body is resilient, and ingenious... the liver and the fatty cells have now been recruited into manufacturing testosterone.

Also the cancer cells have themselves set up internal testosterone manufacturing plants.

(*Life – hah, ya just can't stop it*)

So now we have three sources of food for the cancer that need to be shut down...

When PSA level rises to 2, two new drugs will be administered on top of the one I'll still be on = three drugs.

Rise is expected soon so we will be doing six weekly blood tests to monitor movement.

Chance of stopping the progress is 80% - 20% not.

Hang on to your hats, friends.

The ride might get a bit ugly from here...

Looking forward to update in six weeks

Thank you for your thoughts and prayers...

But I'd prefer you send money to assist in further research into prostate cancer and don't waste your words on me...

I urge you to...

Use your words on your male family members over forty. Early detection brings a 93% chance of survival.

Latest science says that this cancer is a function of your genetic make-up. Which means: it's not diet or activity-related, it doesn't matter who you are or where you come from, or what you eat for dinner. If it decides you're next baby... You're it.

Get the bastard early.

Get checked bi-annually.

Statistically by age 100% of the men who make it to age one hundred will get prostate cancer.

Nine men die in Australia every day from Man Gland cancer.

So if you're planning a long life,

Get your Man Gland checked.

If not for yourself do it for your wife... a broken man gland's not much fun for anyone.

Donate and get info at

www.pcfa.org.au

I have been certified as an ambassador for the PCFA.

So I am qualified to advise and talk on prostate related topics. Feel free to give my details to anyone who had any questions about their Man Gland or anyone who's dealing with a use by date.

I am also available to address groups with a 20 min talk on looking after your Man Gland...

I can do this online or in person.

Funding is available from PCFA to provide transport and accommodation for an Ambassador to address your group... or loved one...

Chapter 9 - Grandma's Favourite Recipes... Busting Mythical Cancer 'Cures'

Sally

During the six years since Tony was first diagnosed, we have heard from so many people of the latest fad that can 'cure' cancer. Messages and emails nearly daily with the 'newest cure' and 'it only costs this much'.

The amount of time to explore everything on Google under the heading of 'cancer' would both be a full-time occupation as well as it costing all your superannuation.

Witch doctors, quacks, and crackpots

The first thing we do when we hear of any new therapy, treatment or product which claims to cure cancer is to research it to see if there are any scientific results to support these claims. If (as in most cases) there isn't any supporting evidence we do not give it another thought, as we believe it is just 'chasing rabbits down holes'.

I, as Tony's carer, went through a phase of listening to anyone who knew anyone who had cancer wanting to know how they had survived it. Clutching at any hope as I imagine everyone faced with this disease, either personally dealing with it, or loving and caring for someone facing it does.

I wanted to believe that apricot kernels cure metastasized cancer and that the power of prayer and positive thinking cures it too.

These people are well meaning. We ourselves have had friends that have gone overseas and spent thousands and thousands of dollars to try the latest fandango trial, to find that once the trial had finished, they were much weaker than when they started.

My belief (for what it's worth) is the vitamin C shots, apricot kernels, turmeric etc, may assist in your general health and well-being, but as a cancer cure without scientific evidence? There is no scientific proof that supports any of it.

As a carer, I know there are some beliefs that I hold that Tony doesn't agree with and vice versa.

I believe that stress can affect your immune levels with any disease or illness. I would rather natural therapy than going to a GP for antibiotics and pain killers, but I remind myself that I am not the one with this disease and suffering from the side-effects of the drugs prescribed.

Tony has been open to having fish slapped over his head, he has had a couple of Reiki sessions, loves his massages, has experimented with Magnetic Therapy and Kinesiology.

One thing he has continued to take on a daily basis is a dose of *Body Balance*, which is a multi-vitamin and mineral liquid supplement, though once again not scientifically proven. But he finds when his supply of this product runs out his body and energy levels drop to have him feel like he is running on only two cylinders.

I remember Tony feeling the side effects of Zoladex after the second injection. We looked into placing him on a vegetarian diet, thinking that this lifestyle would assist in Tony's well-being, boosting his immune system whilst dealing with the medication.

When we discussed this with his oncologist, the advice was to have a balanced diet and stay away from extremes as the body's immune system wouldn't be able to deal with any extra stress – that is: detox and missing out on meat.

Tony

Cancer is viewed societally as a mental disease.

Society is focused on having you be 'positive', and one of our pervasive cultural ideals is that a 'positive' attitude can to cure cancer. Success (a cure) is seen as a personal phenomenon as though one cured oneself by belief, by mind over matter, by sheer will and not by medicine and science.

Cancer has zero interest in beliefs... cancer cannot believe.

I have zero interest in the beliefs of cancer quacks.

The medical industry may be on the wrong track - however, they have a 93 percent verifiable documented success rate of keeping alive men with prostate cancer.

I have found zero documented verifiable statistics on the keeping alive rate of the so-called alternative cancer industry.

What I see is a few aggrieved people striking back at an unforgiving universe, feeding on the misery and the gullibility of humans when their life is threatened. It has occurred to me on many occasions to vent my anger at the very people who are charged with keeping me walking on this planet by joining the noisy band of life-desiring desperate humans.

I am a life-desiring desperate human being; I want to believe that a cure is available as much as I want a god to wave his magic wand to fix me.

But what is, is what is...

Cancer has a self-survival interest...

Cancer will kill its host in search of its survival...

Cancer continues until food source or host is gone...

Cancer will live forever if food source is available...

Cancer does not atrophy and die like we humans.

And being faced with death...

As predicted by statistics of the death rate of men who have succumbed to this disease.

I choose death,

With all its machinations intact.

I choose it all.

I choose love for my community.

I choose fact over hearsay.

I choose aliveness for every day that I get to live.

I choose heartache.

I choose regret.

I choose more heartache.

I choose, I choose, I choose...

I choose to side with persons who willingly put their theories to a panel of experts for examination for facts and efficacy.

That is the facts

No belief required

CHAPTER 10 – CANCER MYTHS

If you, or someone close to you, is dealing with cancer, I can pretty much guarantee that you've gone to Google, and googled cancer. And Google will cheerfully tell you that it has returned 1,080,000,000 results. (that number will likely be bigger tomorrow, because people post things all the time....)

So – how do you work out what to look at? What is useful, true information, and what isn't? Especially when much of what is out there is at best inaccurate, or at worst dangerously misleading (like deadly dangerous...).

Step 1 – apply a big dose of common sense.

Step 2 – See if you can find a paper in a reputable scientific publication (a hospital, a research organisation, a peer reviewed scientific journal etc etc) which agrees with any information you found on a blog, or a discussion site, or similar.

Step 3 – see just how many reputable places you can find which agree on that piece of information.

Step 4 – apply another big dose of common sense.

If you've done that, you just might have found some real information.

Because this book is all about helping you, I thought I'd include some information here, debunking some of the worst / more dubious myths that are circulating. I recommend that you still do your own research, to help you understand the truth of the thing you are dealing with, but this chapter should at least help, by letting you know somethings you can ignore.

Here is a list of myths (not an exhaustive list, but most of the more prevalent ones are listed), each with a bit of information about why they are wrong. At the end of this chapter, you'll also find a list of links to some online sources which go into far more detail about cancer myths.

The Myths

1. Cancer is a man-made, modern disease

No – not by a long way. Cancer has been found, by archaeologists and associated researchers, in skeletons estimated to be at least 3000 years old! In medical texts right throughout history, there are references to damaging growths on the body, and in the body, described as 'canker' since before the year 1000.

In this modern era, we are more aware of cancer, and better equipped with technology to discover it earlier – which makes it seem more prevalent to us – but it is certainly not a modern invention.

Modern lifestyle choices (like smoking) can make a person more likely to get cancer, but equally, it is now known that about 15% of cancers are caused by naturally occurring viruses and bacteria.

2. Antiperspirants or deodorants can cause breast cancer

To date, there is no conclusive evidence to say that antiperspirants, or chemicals contained in them, cause any kind of cancer. There is a lot of supposition out there, which lays blame on these products for causing all sorts of ills (not just cancer), but it is based on anecdotal 'evidence' not on science. So – if the idea concerns you, choose a product which doesn't contain whatever chemicals worry you. But be assured that no study has found a direct link between deodorant and cancer.

3. Superfoods prevent cancer

Sadly, no. To begin with, the concept of a 'superfood' is a thing created by marketers of diet plans and supplements. In reality, whilst there are certainly foods which are healthier than others, and which contain excellent amounts of various necessary nutrients, there is no magic list of foods which have super powers.

A balanced diet of healthy foods will do far more for your health, and your body's ability to deal with anything which threatens your health, than an overindulgence in any one or two specific foods.

4. Cancer has a sweet tooth and people who have cancer shouldn't eat sugar, or sweeteners since they can cause cancer to grow faster.

This one is a distortion of the truth. There is no specific path by which a sugary thing you eat is directed specifically to feed a cancer cell. Every sweet thing you eat, and every carbohydrate you eat, is broken down in your digestive system into various types of 'sugars'. And every cell in your body uses those sugars to burn for energy. Without those sugars, your body can't function. But – cancer cells grow very fast, and, as a consequence, they need more sugars for energy than your other cells do.

So it certainly makes sense to eat a healthy diet, which is balanced, and not overloaded with sugary foods, but still contains some sugar and carbs – that way, your body has all of the nutrients it needs to operate – including the sugars that power your healthy cells. There are different types of sugars, and of sugar substitutes, and some are far worse for your body than others (for example, high fructose corn syrup is broken down in the body via the same pathway that alcohol is, and can, like alcohol, do horrible damage to your liver) – but none of them specifically feed cancer cells above any other cell.

5. Chlorinated water – either drinking water, or pool water you swim in, causes cancer.

This myth comes from the concept that chlorine is always bad for you – which it is, in large concentration – ingest enough, or breath enough chlorine gas, and you will suffer damage and potentially death. But in drinking water, the concentration of chlorine is generally below 1 mg/litre, and in swimming pool water it is generally below 3 mg / litre. Studies over many years have found no negative effects from this concentration. In drinking water in particular, chlorine plays a very important role, by killing bacteria and viruses which may be in the water. This disinfecting action is critical to ensuring clean water supplies (especially in developing countries and rural areas). Chlorinated swimming fools should also have good filters, because the only faint possibility of association between chlorine and cancer is actually via the by-products of chlorine interaction with organic matter in the pool water – and even that association is very weak. If your pool has a good filter, and the chlorine concentration is maintained correctly, you should not be in any way concerned.

6. Cancer is a fungus – and sodium bicarbonate is the cure

It is not known where this idea originally came from – but wherever it was, it wasn't based on science. Some people have suggested this with the theory that people with a candida fungal problem are more likely to have cancer – which is not true. And candida itself is a fungus that is present in almost everyone – it only becomes a problem when the balance in the body is destabilized, and it becomes an overgrowth. That overgrowth can cause a collection of unpleasant symptoms – but it doesn't cause cancer.

The sodium bicarbonate concept is just plain dangerous. High doses of sodium bicarbonate can lead to serious issues, and even death – and whilst neutralizing the acidity of the environment immediately around a cancer cell can help to kill it (in the lab, at least), injecting sodium bicarbonate is not the way to achieve that. Scientists are investigating whether there is any practical way to use sodium bicarbonate to help, without horrible side effects, but so far, there is no evidence to support any use.

7. There's a miracle cancer cure... ...and Big Pharma/ government/ medical associations are suppressing it

This is probably the biggest myth of all, and the most prevalent.

Search for 'miracle cancer cure' or the like, and you will get thousands of results, touting things from the improbable to the dangerous, involving every substance you can think of. But if you dig a bit, you'll find no reputable scientific support for the claims, which are mostly anecdotal - 'Joe did this, and a miracle happened'. The problem with that, is that you are not Joe. Your stage of cancer, type of cancer, underlying health conditions, life history and more, are all different from his, and will all influence how your body reacts to anything and everything. Additionally, when an advocate of an alternative 'cure' promotes it, they only tell you about the people they believe were 'cured' – but how many thousand other people did that, and were not cured?

You can't know that – so you can't assess whether that 'treatment' might have even a fragment of a chance of doing anything helpful for you, or, indeed, whether it might be directly harmful for you.

Most reputable oncologists will be happy to discuss with you whether any alternative approaches you'd like to try may be a helpful addition to standard treatment – but they are not likely to suggest that you abandon conventional care in the hope of a miracle.

With respect to 'Big Pharma' repressing a miracle, aided and abetted by government and medical associations, you need to look at this in terms of practical economics.

Governments would love to have less cancer sufferers occupying hospital beds (so less costs), and doctors would love to have better ways to treat people who are suffering. And whilst it is undoubtedly true (especially in the USA) that manufacturers of drugs make substantial profits from cancer treatments as things are now, you can be certain that, if a treatment which was effective had been found, even in natural products, they would find a way to extract the active ingredient and concentrate it, in a manner which was patentable and able to be profited from. Just repressing it is extremely unlikely. In addition, not for profit cancer research bodies are also working on testing and assessing anything which appears to have even the slightest potential for working as a treatment – and they do not have the profit motive ascribed to commercial companies.

By now, if any of these things did really work in a consistent fashion, at least one of them would likely have been pushed towards use by a not for profit research institute. Sadly, so far, nothing has proven to be entirely effective, although some substances have promise in some limited areas. New things are being investigated every day – but once we have something that works, it will be tested massively to prove it, before any claims are made.

8. Microwaving food in plastic containers and wraps releases harmful, cancer-causing substances. Cooking or storing your food in plastic causes cancer

This is another one where science does not support the myth. And where common sense needs to be applied. There are many different types of plastic, with many different chemicals involved in their manufacture. And each type of plastic has a specific intended use.

So – only use plastics labelled food safe and microwave safe in your microwave!

Other plastics might run a risk of melting, and thereby contaminating your food. Also, consider when the plastic container was made – if it is very old, it will potentially contain things which would not be allowed today. Regardless, even if you use the wrong container, and melt it, the chance of it releasing a substance proven to cause cancer is very, very small. Be sensible, and this will never be an issue.

9. Cancer treatment kills more than it cures – and Chemotherapy always has bad side effects

There's no denying that some parts of treatment, like chemotherapy, are not at all pleasant. These things are designed to kill cancer cells – which are tough things! – and will, unavoidably, kill some healthy cells too. There are side effects. Those side effects vary in intensity for each person – they are not universally bad. Each person reacts differently, and for a fair percentage of patients, the side effects are comparatively mild. They are unpleasant – but they are not likely to kill you – whereas the cancer they are tackling is.

Equally, we can't deny the sad fact that the treatments we have do not work for everyone – especially where the patient is at a late stage of cancer before their treatment is started. In some cases, all treatments can do is to prolong life – not achieve a cure. But, on the whole, treatments are quite effective, and becoming more so every year. Once, a cancer diagnosis was regarded as a death sentence – but that is no longer the case. Now, depending on the type of cancer a patient has, up to three quarters of patients are cured. If you dig into the 'horror stories' out there, you'll often find that the examples they quote are from treatments carried out forty and fifty years ago – a far cry from the way treatments are handled today.

So… accept that your treatment may have side effects, but don't assume that they will be terrible. Go into the process with an open mind, and accept that the doctors you are working with will do their best to make you as comfortable as possible, every step of the way.

10. We've made no progress in fighting cancer

Whilst we still have no treatment which is a guaranteed cure, we have made huge strides in fighting cancer. Now, twice as many people survive cancer as did forty years ago. And the rate at which that is improving is accelerating.

But some cancers are harder to beat than others, and have been tougher to find effective treatments for – such as brain, lung, oesophageal and pancreatic cancers – but research continues, and survival rates, even for the difficult ones, are steadily improving.

11. 'Acidic' diets cause cancer

Some myths about cancer are persistent, despite the facts of basic biology. The concept that overly 'acidic' diets cause your blood to become 'too acidic', and thereby increase your risk of cancer is just that kind of myth. People who continue to spread this myth suggest that you increase your intake of healthier 'alkaline' foods like green vegetables and fruits (including, paradoxically, lemons) to change the acidity of your blood.

This is biological nonsense.

It is true that cancer cells can't live in an overly alkaline environment, but neither can any of the other cells in your body. Your blood is normally very slightly alkaline. Each person's might be slightly different, but it will be within a very narrow range. It is kept that way by your kidneys, which achieve that by ensuring that anything extra, outside that range, is eliminated in your urine. So the pH of your urine will change, based on what you have eaten, day by day. But that doesn't mean that your body is either too acidic, or too alkaline – quite the opposite – because the pH of your urine varies like that, your body, and th pH of your blood, stays perfectly in balance.

There is such a thing as acidosis – which can happen when you get seriously ill, or as a result of poisoning, and your kidneys can no longer keep things balanced – but it is not a result of an acidic diet! So – by all means, eat those healthy green veggies, as the proponents of this myth suggest, because, yes, they are good for you, but they are not going to change how 'acidic, or alkaline' your body is – not one bit.

12. Sharks don't get cancer

This myth came about through a tangle of rather long reach extensions from one idea to the next. But before I tell you anything about that, let's just answer the question outright – **yes**, sharks do get cancer. Researchers have found multiple cases of cancer in sharks.

Whilst sharks do seem to have a low rate of cancer, not enough studies have been done to measure exactly how low.

But, if that's the case, where did this myth come from?

It started in the 1970s, when researchers discovered that, if you implanted cartilage next to a tumour, it stopped blood vessels from growing into the tumour area, and thereby starved the tumour. From there, extrapolation set in. Almost the entire skeleton of a shark is composed of cartilage – so they were seen as an excellent source of cartilage for experiments. The next stage of extrapolation came when a doctor came to the very unsubstantiated conclusion that cartilage would limit tumour growth if taken in a pill, rather than being implanted beside the tumour (which it doesn't do at all). From there, he created a big business, selling shark cartilage pills with all sorts of promises of a miracle. The end result? A terrible impact on shark populations, and no effect whatsoever on the cancers of the people who paid for his pills.

So – sharks do get cancer, and shark cartilage won't help cure your cancer at all.

13. Cancer is contagious.

Cancer is most definitely not contagious. People who have cancer very much need to reassurance of the touch of their loved ones, so don't hold back in groundless fear. This myth seems to have arisen because certain viruses (which are contagious), such as human Papilloma virus, and hepatitis B or C, can lead to the development of cancer. There are, in most cases, vaccines available for those viruses – consult your doctor if you are concerned.

14. Coffee, tea, and other hot drinks cause cancer

No – if anything, there is evidence that coffee and tea may provide a slight protective benefit with respect to your risk of cancer. But...

There is some evidence that regularly drinking very, very hot drinks of any kind (including plain hot water) where the drink is at 65 degrees C or more can cause an ongoing irritation of the throat lining, which can lead to cancer.

So – drink whichever beverage you prefer, just don't drink it too hot!

15. Fluoride in water causes cancer

This is still debated by many, but, so far, all studies done on the subject have proven to show either no association between fluoride and cancer, or have been inconclusive. The concentrations in drinking water are very low, and studies have shown that fluoride in water does cause a small reduction in childhood tooth decay. For some people, however, it also leads to white spots on the teeth – which have no negative effect.

16. Cosmetics, including lipsticks, and personal care items like sunscreen, hair dye, talcum powder, shampoo, and toothpaste cause cancer.

There have been many claims made that the chemicals used in many cosmetic items are damaging – but none have yet been substantiated with respect to causing cancer. It is possible that you may be sensitive to one of more constituents used in some cosmetics, but that doesn't make them carcinogenic.

If a product irritates your skin, stop using it, and try an alternative. Each person has different sensitivities. Some ingredients can make your skin more sun sensitive, which can, in turn, make it easier to get sunburned – but it will be the sunburn that puts you at greater risk of skin cancer, not the cosmetics – you should always be aware of how long you have been in the sun, and avoid sunburn.

Lipsticks do contain very small amounts of substances which, in far greater concentration, are dangerous, and may be carcinogenic. But the amounts present in lipstick are so small that it has been determined to present no risk. If the idea of it still worries you, choose lighter coloured lipsticks (the dark ones often use more of the suspect ingredients), or go without lipstick entirely – but really, unless you were actually eating the equivalent of multiple lipsticks a day (rather than just putting a thin layer on your lips), the chances of you being affected in any way are vanishingly small.

Sunscreen – whilst sunscreen does contain nanoparticles of titanium dioxide (TiO2) and zinc oxide (ZnO), these have been determined to be non-carcinogenic, whereas getting sunburned is most definitely going to increase your risk of skin cancer. As with any other product which you apply to your skin, some people will be more sensitive to the ingredients of a product than others – so if a particular sunscreen irritates your skin, try a different one, until you find one that works for you.

Talcum powder – prior to the 1970s, there were a number of cases where Talc was found to be contaminated with asbestos (due to them being mined close to each other quite often). Once this was discovered, stringent rules and processes were put in place to prevent it. Still, the fear of contamination created pre 1970 has persisted, creating this myth. Studies since then have found no link between talc use and cancer.

Toothpaste – pre 2016, toothpastes often contained an antibacterial ingredient called triclosan. Whilst studies have not proven a connection to cancer, concerns have been enough that manufacturers have ceased using it, in general. The quantities in toothpaste are so small, that the chance of an impact is very tiny regardless.

With respect to hair dye, the belief that it may cause cancer comes from the hair dyes used pre 1990 (or perhaps even earlier) which did, in some cases, have ingredients which proved to be slightly carcinogenic. Since 1990 there have been vast improvements in the ingredients used for hair dyes, to the point where, in the last twenty years, no study has been able to find any remaining link between dyes and cancer. So, you can feel safe using modern hair dyes.

17. Some dental fillings cause cancer

The traditional silver coloured dental fillings are made from amalgam – which is compounded of mercury, silver, tin and copper. There has been a lot of concern in recent years that mercury might 'leak' from the fillings into the body – and mercury is known to be carcinogenic. But multiple studies in different parts of the world have identified that the amounts which could 'leak' are vanishingly small, and that amalgam fillings do not present a cancer risk.

Studies have found that there is no evidence that amalgam fillings cause cancer, or have any other adverse health effects. There is the possible risk that amalgam dental fillings can sometimes cause local side effects or allergic reactions in a limited number of people. These hypersensitivity reactions are rare and can be treated by removing the amalgam filling. There are alternatives to amalgam fillings which can be used if you are still concerned about the carcinogenicity of mercury.

However, it is not advised that you remove your current amalgam filling to replace it with another filling, as this can weaken the tooth. If you are concerned, or fear that you are having an allergic reaction to your fillings, discuss your options with your dentist.

But, whilst the filling may be making you uncomfortable, it is not likely to give you cancer.

18. Food additives cause cancer

Most food additives are completely safe, with respect to cancer at least. Some people have sensitivities or allergies to some additives, and should approach foods containing them with caution – not because of a cancer risk, but because of the risk of allergic reaction.

Additives are used in food for one of three reasons - to improve the taste or appearance of a processed food, to improve the keeping quality or stability of a food, or to preserve food when this is the most practical way of extending its storage life.

In recent years, many studies have been done on a wide range of additives, and, whilst quite a few have been found to cause allergic reactions or other undesirable affects in some people, the only one which has been found to have anything approaching the possibility of being carcinogenic, is sodium nitrate or sodium nitrate – which is sometimes used in processed meats as a preservative and colour or flavour enhancer.

So – if you are worried about this, avoid processed meats, and if you do detect an unpleasant reaction t some foods, it is likely a sensitivity which can be managed by avoiding that food – it is very unlikely to ever lead to cancer.

19. Thinking positively can cure cancer

Whilst a positive attitude will undoubtedly help you deal with the challenges of day to day life if you are facing cancer, there is little evidence to link positive thinking to actually beating cancer, any more than there is evidence to link negative thoughts with getting cancer.

Everyone will go through moments of stress and uncertainty in their cancer journey, and there is no right way to feel. I would, however, encourage you to find a balance which lets you feel 'not miserable' as much as possible – simply because it is a lot easier to deal with everything that happens if you can find some joy, somewhere, in your life. Equally, things like meditation can help you cope, because such things have been proven to assist with stress, and releasing tension in the body.

20. Treating a cancer with surgery causes it to spread

This myth comes from the idea that a surgeon might accidentally 'smear some cancer cells on other nearby tissues'.

This is very unlikely – and unlikely to cause a spread of cancer if it happened. But, just to be sure, surgeons take extreme care when taking biopsies, or performing operations to remove cancers, to also take some healthy cells from all around the cancer, so that there is no risk of anything being left to spread.

Not all cancers spread at the same rate, or in the same way, so depending on the type of cancer, surgeons choose methods which optimise the prevention of any risk of spread.

In the end, the option is a simple one – if you leave the cancer there, in most cases it will spread. If you go through surgery to remove it, the chances are far higher that it will be completely removed, than that it will still be able to spread.

The choice is pretty obvious, when you look at it that way.

21. Mobile phones cause cancer

This is another area where there has been much debate. Because high energy radiation is known to be carcinogenic, people tend to worry about all types of radiation. The radiation used by mobile phones to communicate is a very low energy microwave radiation.

Over many years, there have been studies done, some involving following up to 800,000 people, each for ten years or more, which have found no association between mobile phone use and increased cancer risk.

There have also been studies done of people who already had cancers of the head and neck, to attempt, using their memory (which, of course, may be inherently unreliable) to assess how much they had used mobile phones in the twenty years before being diagnosed with cancer. These studies also, with one exception (an area of doubt where the data was not statistically significant, but in which a very faint association seemed to be seen), found no correlation between mobile phone use and cancer.

The only place where the mobile phone networks may produce enough radiation to be at all of concern is very close up to the base stations which link all phones in an area into the network.

These base stations do output much stronger radiation, but the intensity drops off rapidly as you move away from them. As a result, access to the base stations, and the tall towers they are usually mounted on, is generally tightly controlled.

22. Living or working near power lines causes cancer

Similarly to the reasons that people fear the radiation from mobile phones, people have come to fear power lines. The electric and magnetic fields which exist anywhere that electricity is transmitted to cables are extremely low frequency fields. That means that they are very low risk to start with.

Nonetheless, many studies have been done, with fairly consistent results.

Those results have found that there is inadequate evidence to support any link between cancer and the fields associated with power lines, with one exception. There does appear to be a weak link between prolonged and intense exposure to magnetic fields, and an increased risk of childhood leukaemia.

To receive that sort of exposure, a person would need to pretty much live immediately beside a big electrical substation or similar.

So – if this worries you, choose your house location to be away from big electrical installations – but you need not, based on all current evidence, fear normal power lines in your district.

23. Stress causes cancer

This myth is pretty pervasive. But it is another case where the link is not there – not directly, anyway. When we are stressed, we tend to do things which are not good for us – whether that is not exercising, not eating a healthy diet, smoking too much, drinking too much, or something similar. And some of those choices can lead us to a higher risk of cancer – especially things like smoking!

So, whilst stress does not directly cause cancer, it can certainly be a contributing factor in making it harder for your body to deal with cancer. In addition, when we are stressed, we tend to be tense, physically – and all of that tension in the body can lead to muscle pain and the like.

So – reducing your stress levels is a great way to help you stay healthy, even if being stressed is not a direct cause of cancer.

Links to sites with more information:

Each of these links will take you to information about cancer myths, in far more detail that I have covered here. Many of these sites then also link out the reports of the specific scientific studies they reference, so that you can read even more detail if you wish to.

http://www.bbc.co.uk/news/science-environment-26627941

https://scienceblog.cancerresearchuk.org/2014/03/24/dont-believe-the-hype-10-persistent-cancer-myths-debunked/

https://www.mayoclinic.org/diseases-conditions/cancer/in-depth/cancer-causes/art-20044714

https://www.cancerwa.asn.au/resources/cancermyths/

https://www.cancer.org.au/content/about_cancer/factsheets/employers/Cancer_myths_and_facts_fact_sheet_April%202017.pdf

https://www.cancercenter.com/community/blog/2019/02/11-cancer-myths-busted

https://www.bupa.com.au/healthlink/conditions-and-treatments/medical-condition-and-disease/cancer/living-with-cancer-and-beyond/debunking-cancer-myths

https://www.singaporecancersociety.org.sg/learn-about-cancer/cancer-basics/cancer-myths-debunked.html

Chapter 11 - True Life Extenders

Sally

Why Bother ...

When faced with the news that without treatment, Tony's life expectancy would be 6-12 months, and with treatment up to 3 years, we had a choice to make. Tony was 54 not 84. Tony had so much life still to experience; he hadn't had his nine lives yet. We had a discussion about going on the suggested treatment, but at no stage did I think Tony wouldn't do the treatment. I also believed that it would extend his life. If it did work, that would allow an extended 3 years. At the time, to me, it was a no-brainer - I understood that this meant a radical treatment plan as his PSA level was extremely high and the cancer had spread into his kidney and liver areas.

With research developing all the time who knows what treatment could be available in a couple of years. Yes, the treatment is keeping Tony alive and along with that he deals with the side effects. On the plus side, currently Tony's last injection was nine months ago, and yes, the PSA level is rising slowly but at least it's not an injection every three months.

Tony's cholesterol rose when he first commenced treatment, so the doctor put him on cholesterol medication to assist it artificially. We cut down the saturated fats in our diets which assisted his levels a little bit. Tony decided not to take the cholesterol tablets while we were overseas in Thailand recently. Instead, he cut his meals to smaller portions and began eating every 3 hours - mainly protein, vegetables, and rice (and a lot of chilli).

When we returned a month after this change in diet, his cholesterol level had come down. Some say stress, diet and exercise contribute and impact on high cholesterol levels. He changed all these in that one month.

I personally think as a carer, a true 'life extender' is a combination of a balanced mind and body approach, in other words going into a diet that is extreme will deplete the body of its nutrients which would potentially stress the mind.

Everything in moderation

Of course it is proven scientifically that if you eat junk food all day your body's organs will be put under gigantic pressure causing potential sickness and other diseases.

I have observed when Tony is taking on a lot which may not be aligned to what he is up to in life, he becomes stressed, not just by mood but also his outlook in life. He has become overwhelmed with 'having to' complete deadlines, he then wants to chuck it all in and not do anything.

We have aimed to maintain balance with both mental and physical exercise and importantly for him to be kind to himself.

Tony

Bring love of the Game of Life to life

Today is the first day of the best of my life... it is the best day I have yet to see...

Tomorrow may be better but it can never match the sheer brilliance of this day that I am experiencing...

The moments of today are the foundations of our tomorrows.

Bring hunger for love of the game of life to today simply for the opportunity of experiencing the joy of being alive.

Take this moment as you read this to experience.... No goals, no ambition, nowhere to get...

Nothing to fix.

Just be right where you are with who you are and how you are... and how you say they are...

That, my friend, is the place to be.

Come join me in playing this thing we call life for no other reason than you can... now that the day has passed I make ready for another day where I shall awake as a human and get up and go to work at avoiding being human for the whole day until I shall make this same pledge again.

It's ma bitday!

Fifty-five years ago ma bits discharged onto this planet.

What a ride!!!

I've had love, success, disease, sickness, health, lived well, crashed, woken up in hospital 3 times; I've challenged mother nature many times, fought bushfires, fought friends, fought enemies, fought myself... been bankrupt; moved interstate (six times), moved home (about 27 times).....

Had one truly amazing bitching gorgeous wife, many lovers, three children, three sisters, four brothers, a beautiful mother... good times, bad times, some truly amazing times.

I've painted, plastered, meditated; sold stuff, sold more stuff, bought stuff; been to Europe, Fiji, Thailand, Cairns; had about 100 cars, had motorcycles (& broken bones).

And for all this I am thankful for all time.

I've even changed my horoscope from Sagittarius to Cancerian.

Thank you to those who cared for me and thank you to those who couldn't give a rat's about me; may each of you get everything you want in life and then some.

Because fifty-five years on - that's what I have to show for all of it: awesome memories, awesome family and awesome friends.

My Identity Doesn't Have Cancer

Cancer maybe hanging on some of my tubes but it ain't hanging on me. I don't have cancer, my body does, and until my body says stop I'm a going for it.

'For what?' I hear you ask?

Living each day open, free, powerfully... punch-drunk on life. I'm writing a book focused at empowering Cancerians in living powerfully, punch-drunk on life.

It's about having a use-by date stamped on your life ticket....

It's about playing life with the cards you've been dealt....

It's about being cool with that...

It's about dealing with the despair you have for your long-lost future...

CHAPTER 12 – FISCAL-NESS

Sally

Home Management... Time Management... Money Management

Once you're past the initial shock, you realise that you still have to deal with the ordinary, day-to-day things: finances, jobs, household chores, etc.

In my case, I was working fulltime AND managing a household. Added to that were the jobs that Tony could no longer manage. So I researched the types of assistance we were eligible for, and how to apply for them.

I'd never gone to a bank to see what options we had. I was surprised at just how much help is out there if you know where to look. I'll share with you exactly what I did, that really took the pressure off our finances and kept the income coming in. (This works even if your insurance cover is inadequate or non-existent)

In the lull before the storm, Tony was able to keep working for a couple of months after the first injection of Zoladex. Then bang, he would wake up about 10 am then get to the job by 12 midday, stuffed at 3 pm and back home asleep by 4 pm. The treatment was at work, hence the muscle weakness had commenced.

My initial reaction, I think, was selfish: 'How am I going to maintain our lifestyle if we only have one income?' I certainly went into practical mode, first working out our budget, as we hadn't had one prior to this. Tony was self-employed with no insurance to cover his inability to earn money and no superannuation.

Firstly, we went through the paperwork involved in applying for a Centrelink benefit, a disability pension as Tony's expected life span was limited at that stage. Fortunately, I was very familiar with this procedure as it was within my field of employment. Understanding this system makes it a lot simpler.

Tony made an appointment with the first urologist who diagnosed him. He completed the necessary paper work, stressing that the cancer was stage 4 and had spread to other organs, his life expectancy and that symptoms were going to be ongoing more than 24 months. This pension enabled Tony to get a pension card for cheaper medication and bulk-billing at the GP's. What it didn't do was provide us with much money per fortnight, try just over $200.

My income was too high!!! It certainly wasn't high enough to afford our weekly expenditures. I was pretty ruthless with the budget; it's amazing how much you spend without accountability and how much you can live off when you have to. Here's where I found myself ringing utility companies to go on set payments - these simple calls saved us over $300 a month. I made an appointment with the bank manager to discuss consolidating loans to one payment, which also enabled us to pay out our credit cards.

I became creative with shopping and meals. I discovered that I could apply for 'hardship' which allowed a minimum payment for up to six months with some of the debts. I shopped at food banks and discount outlets, saving heaps. We were on borderline breaking even, living week to week. A lot has happened since those initial days. When Tony's health enables it, he can work the odd day or two, adding this income to our holiday budget. We have had the opportunity to have some awesome holidays, as we have found that it is imperative to our well-being to tick experiences of a lifetime off your list.

These simple things also began a habit pattern for what came along in 2016. I needed major surgery on my ankle to address a long-term genetic issue, estimating that I would be non weight-bearing for eight weeks. I organised that I would work from home, no dramas. A week after I had the operation, the company I worked for went into voluntary liquidation. The fortunate fall back was I had taken insurance through my superannuation three years previously which supplied us with 75% of the income I was on. Suddenly we found ourselves in a financial situation where we were no longer able to find money to service the credit card debt we had. I researched the options for what we could do, including stalling payments and applying for hardship to decrease the monthly amount to pay.

Upon ringing one of the banks, I learnt that I could apply for waiving the debt off the card due to our circumstances. I completed a financial statement, medical forms for each of us, supplied bank statements etc and found that the banks would waive our debt without a black mark on our name.

This has been a huge relief.

The Bucket List

The majority of the population are not aware of how long they have left with their loved ones!

When someone who is very close to you is provided a timeline there is an urgency in the sense of 'how do we prioritise the time we have left, what is important to us with the time we have been given?'

For Tony, it was asking each of us to provide a list of five things which we would like to do with him individually. For me it was spending time enjoying the simple things we enjoyed doing together like walking on the beach and going on holidays.

The children were all different with their wishes.

At first it was challenging for them to get their heads around the request - for example, one of the things our eldest chose was for Tony to teach him more about the mechanics of a car, and it was great for them to fix a boat trailer together.

I think every family should undertake this invaluable task, though it was uncomfortable to write down, as at the time we found ourselves thinking we are all fine, we spend time with Dad/ Tony all the time. This put another slant on it, that life is too short, no matter how old you are. I believe we as a family are a lot more open in saying what needs to be said.

Another priority was for Tony to leave a legacy to his family, in the form of this book and his thoughts on life, living and death. This ties in with his passion for assisting people going through similar journeys. He also became an ambassador for the Prostate Foundation. This involves educating groups of men and their partners.

Tony is also a convener at a monthly prostate support group which meets once a month. This is a group for men of all ages to attend to hear about the latest procedures available as well as gaining support from others. New men to the group, who have not shared their news with anyone (including their family!), come along for the first time - often releasing stress with tears as they have felt that the 'manly' thing to do was to try and cope with all the mental and physical elements of this disease by themselves.

Tony encourages people to take life on in spite of the disease. He accomplishes this every day and I for one know that this is a huge legacy.

We learnt very early on not to sweat the small stuff, and it's all small stuff. This attitude has certainly assisted us through the six years of this roller coaster ride and our experiences with our family and friends.

Tony

Fear of Success

Fear of success is myth. It's a story lodged in our minds that we use as a looking-good mask...

'Fear' (being afraid) is not *fear... fear* is only present when physical life is endangered. *Fear* is like panic-running from a knife attack... and then it's actually a hi-jack fuelled by instinct... *to seize possession or control*

'Fear' is more or less superstition.

Fear is distinguishable by noting that it controls you regardless of your thoughts about what's going on - you're running and wondering, 'why?!!'

What you've described is reaction to an event in your past that is re-enacted by today's events. This is normal human animal behaviour. We are designed for survival only. We are not designed for success except as survival is a success.

Modern day success is a man-made invention. It is foreign to our instinctive nature. That's why we make up stories around our success (and fearing success), in order to look good to a world that we think requires our success to further our survival in society.

And when that success doesn't happen, we make up more stories about why it didn't happen. You are forced to exist as a human in a society that dictates being other than naturally human

If you want success then know it will always occur as foreign... during and at the end of that road that you choose to travel.

And you are just as valuable to society as any of the 'most societally successful' humans that walk this earth...

Chapter 13 - Cramming 30 Years into 3 Years

Tony

At age 46 my business career came to a halt due to illness... (eventually diagnosed as celiac disease). And now at age 56 it occurs to me that terminal cancer diagnosis... is Interrupting my return to my career!

I find myself making plans, as I always have, setting targets, designing a business future that will provide occupation and income. The most recent one plotted growing my consultancy business to a level of $5,000 per week in income, and includes plans to build my dream future.... Who programmed me to this?

At the age of 5, I invented that the context of my life has been, 'you don't care about me and I don't care about you'. For sharing with my younger brothers what I had learned at school that day about sex, I was chastised by my mother and beaten by my father.

I see now that 'you don't care about me' translates as *life* doesn't care about me. I also see now how that has played into my life. In my relationships and in my career pursuits, it shows up as...

I am a has-been, was once pretty cool (if I say so myself), but now I'm cooked...

I apologize for selling out on you in my need for appreciation and for stepping over what was there to be said, afraid that what I had to say wouldn't make the grade or make a difference.

Love is... taking actions that add to the quality and context of the life of another human.

My New Year Resolutions...

I resolve to lose forever the identity that I invested 50-odd years inventing; I resolve from now to be human only. To never again hold that there is a me, or a you; I choose life now exactly as it is. Free of any and all expectation, I am free and I am welded to my humanity as are you. I choose this for the pure joy of playing the game of life.

For no other reason than the opportunity to experience once again the child-like sheer joy of being in love with this thing we call life, please refer to me now by my new nickname 'HB', short for Human Being.

Consulting business three days per week and one morning to attend networking marketing function,

1 day per week Tony time, 3 days a week off = no business activity Saturday, Sunday, Monday.

Day 547 - Ready to roll with whatever is there ...

Morning is complete.

I am complete.

Holidays and life with money 'Living the Dream' starts here until whenever if ever.

Chapter 14 - The Primeval Urge to Survive

Tony

For nearly two decades I have engaged and been engaged by the thought-twisting and thought–provoking conceptions employed by *Landmark Worldwide*, a self-awareness education company. I first attended what they call 'The Landmark Forum' 18 years ago (2001). It opened me up to realizing a lot of stuff about why I do things the way I do them. Here I am sharing with you my take on some of the stuff that I have learnt about whilst attending some of Landmark's courses. Since I attended that course and many others, and got more involved with the company, I have been dedicated to pursuing what makes me tick, and providing the opportunity, out of pure love, to others to take on investigating their own thought processes to be free of self-imposed constraints. This is called 'enrolment' – enrolment in life and enrolment in YOU.

In the Landmark Forum, Landmark proposes that...

'You can have anything you want for yourself and your life, that you invent as a possibility and enrol others in your having gotten.'

Enrolment

Enrolment is a two-step process that naturally occurs when you

1. Share an insight with others about a past way of being that you have identified and
2. You then share with them a new possibility that you have invented about how you would like them to view you from now on.

You know if enrolment is present if the person with whom you have shared it is left moved, touched, or inspired by what you have shared.

'Enrolment' calls for bringing that which currently exists but is hidden from your world into your view, the thing existed all along but was located in a bind spot. ie: it was there but you couldn't see it. It is a process by which you can take on new things that become possible for you to see and do, whereas prior to enrolment the possibility of you having the thing you said you wanted in your life did not exist...

Because prior to having an enrolment conversation, that idea or thing you desired was held inside your head only. If it only existed inside your head... It has zero existence out in the real world.

When you release it to the world by expressing it to others, it begins to take shape and substance in the world that is outside of you (i.e. in others)... and when you have others identifying with you as your new possibility and observing you operating in that new possibility they react in a new way toward you.

Why have I told you about enrolment? Because with enrolment anything that you want for your life becomes possible...

A breakthrough I had during one of Landmark's seminars...

At age seven, I saw that I had created 'that people were bastards and I should not engage with them or they might cause bad things for me'.

I saw that I had at age seven a vivid memory of my mother walking out of our home, saying she wasn't coming back. I recalled that I chased her up the street. I asked her what was wrong, what did I do, and she said, 'it's not just you; it's all of you' (I had 5 brothers and sisters at that time). In that moment the seven-year old me invented that I didn't cause her to leave, so it must have been them, my brothers and sisters and they have made my mum run away and they were all bastards. This translated (as I grew older and collected more evidence for the position) that all people are bastards, don't trust 'em at all because if you do, they will run away.

At the same time, seven-year old me invented that I had to walk on eggshells around my mother in case I did something that would make her run away again.

Prior to this seminar, I wasn't aware that I had an 'all people are bastards' story running in my brain. I thought it was the truth, that people really are bastards. I didn't understand that it was a story that I invented when I was seven years old.

Now that I have seen that I made this up I was able to look at what it has brought to, and kept, from my life... I was also able to choose to give up that way of being and invent a new way of being and have that new way of being be present in my life.

My new possibility is being open in communication with all people and that all people freely communicate in harmonious ways.

> ...That all people feel valued and loved and cherished by all the other humans on the planet
>
> ...That there isn't a place I can't go that won't welcome me or mine, be that place real or imagined

I used to see relationships as a tool, a tool to be used only to get somewhere or something. Through an exercise that I participated in at a Landmark relationship seminar, I saw that at age seven I invented how I relate to people.

The new possibility I have invented is that I love all people and all of their contributions to the world. I love all people for being exactly who they are and for being exactly who they are not.

For I see that who you are for me is controlled by me, and only me, and that you have nothing to do with how I choose that I see you or relate to you.

Even if you yell or scream or shoot me down...

You are still a magnificent human being.

Some other Landmark stuff...

Integrity

Integrity is honouring my word and having my word be how it goes.

Having my word be how the day and the circumstances of the day go.

Integrity is my honouring only a way of being which supports how I said it would go.

When I'm not living from a created context that I have individually created, I am out of integrity and out of power to command anything to go as I say.

Only Integrity delivers personal power. Where there is no integrity there is no power in the present, nor is there any power available to be had in the future.

The "IT" .... Your identity?

(IT = Your Brain and Identity)

IT does not give a F*@k about what I or we say we want...

IT is programmed to survive everything. IT is programmed to restrict you from entering places and spaces where IT considers things might not go well...

IT is programmed to survive and destroy even the simplest spurt toward success...

The IT will disregard all and everything IT considers a challenge to ITs survival... (IT considers survival as keeping what already is in place in the same place)

The IT will create and give what seem like valid reasons and justifications for not proceeding with the plans or possibilities that (you as possibility) have instructed IT to carry out...

IT will kick and scream and complain argue, blame, justify, scheme, and resolve to cause you to stop you making IT do stuff IT doesn't want to do.

IT doesn't want to do new stuff... IT wants to do safe old stuff that has been tested to contain no chance of not surviving.

As soon as you give IT instructions to do some future-based activity, where ITs survival may be threatened... IT turns you and has you legging it the other way.

The solution...

Let IT do ITs thing, whilst you stand firm and command IT to do your thing...

The thing you were inspired to do...

Before IT took your inspiration away...

IT is the true dream stealer – it was not your neighbour/ Aunt/ Brother or Uncle who stole your dream ... Your IT stole your own dream.

Now that you know that's what you did go get your dream out, dust it off and instruct IT to carry out your demand to realize your dream.

And be ready for ITs excuses, reasons, justifications, arguments against and general silly carry on.

Tell IT the longer IT refuses to carry out your plans the longer IT will have to fight you for control of your bodily actions.

Whilst noting IT will fight you tooth and nail every step of the way until you realize your dream and then IT will tell you it wasn't worth it. It's right, IT is not worth arguing with...

Tell IT what to do and how to be. Give IT regular doses of possibility...

IT has that *possibility* is a scary place...

In the past I was not interested in communicating and sharing with people about what goes on for me in my head. As a result of a lesson at Landmark's Relationship Course I got to see that at age seven I decided all people are bastards and I don't talk to them.

So having seen that, for forty-five years that's how I've operated, I've chosen to change that.

My new way of being is...

Love and Communication.

So, Bastards... here is the communication...

I offer you the opportunity to contribute and come along for the RIDE with me as I grind this Cancer Bastard into the ground, sliding and kicking and kicking its head... until me or it is dead.

CHAPTER 15 - GETTING YOUR AFFAIRS IN ORDER

Sally

Faced with the potential of Tony's life being cut short, we were plunged into the land of conversations about wills, life Insurance, funeral insurance, and funeral arrangements. In our situation, our will was 27 years old, pre- children, a lifetime ago.

Life Insurance

We both had life insurance with funeral expenses built in. Tony's life insurance had a 'terminal illness payout' component in it, which in essence meant that if the oncologist deemed the terminal illness to decrease life expectancy to 12 months or less, the insurance under-writers would consider this to be eligible for a pay out of the life insurance.

It is important that you have nominated beneficiaries in the life insurance policy (these can be changed at any time), so your insurance pay-out is not held up in probate.

Steps for Getting Your Affairs in Order

It's a good idea for everyone to get their affairs in order, whether you have cancer or not. By preparing a few simple documents, you can make sure that your wishes are followed, and you will make things easier for your family at a difficult time.

'Getting your affairs in order' usually means:

- making a will
- preparing documents that will help others to make decisions for you if you're not able to make them yourself
- •nominating a beneficiary for your superannuation and insurance
- sorting out legal and financial paperwork

If you or a partner is facing shortened life expectancy, there are some questions you may need to ponder:

Firstly, do you have an updated will? There are many options in updating your will or preparing a will. You can organise it through your solicitor or alternatively DIY kits are available (although these are pretty basic in my opinion).

All adults should have a valid will. It's the best way to make sure that your assets are distributed in the way you would like after you die.

Why is it important to make a will?

Even if you don't own much, making a will is a good idea. Having a will makes it easier for your family and friends to make legal and financial arrangements after you die.

Without a will, these arrangements can be complicated and expensive. A will is particularly important for anyone with a family or dependants, especially if you are separated or divorced.

Things to consider when setting or updating a will

You may want to consider leaving part of your estate to a charitable organisation.

How will your estate be shared amongst your beneficiaries?

Who will you appoint as executor(s) for your will?

Who should look after your children if you and the other parent both die before the youngest child turns 18 (guardians)?

Do you want to nominate an amount of maintenance for your children?

Do you want to give other directions, such as preference of burial or cremation, or plan your funeral in advance?

Do you need to consider planning for your estate?

For example, do you

- Want to pass on a family business;
- Have a superannuation payout;
- Want to give a gift to charity;
- Have capital losses;
- Have life insurance;
- Have debts to be paid out;
- Want flexibility in distributing your assets, for example, there are more children or grandchildren on the horizon.
- Where will you put your will? Have you told anyone? E.g. The executor, where is the will located?
- Do you want to arrange and pay for your funeral in advance?

Making a will

A will is a legal document that records what you want to happen to your assets after you die. These assets are called your estate. Anyone aged 18 or older can make a will, as long as they have 'testamentary capacity'. This means that they:

- understand what a will is
- can communicate what they want to put in their will and why.

If there could be any doubt about whether you have testamentary capacity (for example, if you are on heavy pain medication that is affecting how you think), it's a good idea to get a doctor's certificate. Who should make a will? If you don't make a will, the law will decide who gets your property when you die, and it might not be who you would like.

How do I make a will?

There are a number of ways to make a will. A lawyer can help you draft a will. Some people draft their own wills using kits bought from a newsagency or post office. However, there are certain requirements for a will to be valid and using a lawyer ensures you get it right. Lawyers charge different fees to draft wills.

Ask around to make sure you get the best deal. If you can't afford to pay, Cancer Council may be able to arrange a lawyer to draft a will for free.

Where should I keep my will? Keep your will in a safe place. Your lawyer will usually hold the will for you, or you could keep it with your other important documents. It's important you tell your executor where your will is kept.

It's a good idea to review a will regularly (e.g. every five years) to see if it needs updating. If you have been married since you made a will, you will need to make a new will. If you have been divorced, separated, or had children since your last will, it may be a good idea to write a new will or have your lawyer help you make a formal addition called a codicil.

Can anyone challenge my will? Yes.

The law expects people to make 'proper provision' for certain people. These include:

- Current and former spouses
- De facto partners who are living with you around the time of your death
- Children
- Financially dependent grandchildren
- Any other financially dependent people in your household
- Any person who is living with you in a close personal relationship at the time of your death.

If you don't make provisions for these people, they can go to court and challenge your will. The Court will consider their needs, their relationship to you and whether they contributed to your estate (e.g. as part of a marriage). If you want to leave any of these people out of your will, you should talk to a lawyer.

What happens if I don't make a will?

An administrator (often a relative) will be appointed to carry out similar duties to an executor. The law provides a formula for the distribution of assets of a person who has not left a will. This may not work out the way you would have wanted. If you don't have a will, legal procedures may be more complicated and time-consuming.

Advance health care directive

An advance health care directive is a document that sets out your wishes for your future medical care. This is sometimes called a living will. Types of issues it covers – Whether you want to receive artificial nutrition or hydration, whether you want to be resuscitated, or whether you want to receive antibiotics as part of your treatment. The more guidance you provide on your preferences, the more likely your family and health care providers will make decisions that respect your wishes.

If you have particular religious beliefs that impact on your health care decisions, you can also record these in your advance health care directive.

Superannuation death benefit nominations

When a member of a superannuation fund dies, the fund pays out their death benefit to one or more of their dependants. This includes the preserved amount (the contributions the member made while they were working) and any insurance benefit. You can tell your superannuation fund who you would like to receive your death benefit.

Organising your paperwork

It's a good idea to have all of your paperwork in the one place. This will make it easier if, for example, you need to be in hospital for a long time and a family member has to help you with financial and legal matters.

Important documents to gather together might include:

- Birth, marriage, and divorce certificates
- Bank and credit card information
- Share and other investment details
- Centrelink and Medicare details
- Superannuation and insurance information
- Funeral information
- House title / lease documents
- Passport

CHAPTER 16 - ZACKERY

Tony

Existentially....

Today in the midst of contemplating death I have contemplated what life is about...

Today I offer you these rants -

Today I am in the same position as every human on this planet.

Today I exist (I think).

Today I am a *tube* that lives on a planet somewhere in a cosmos of galaxies, created by I know not what, or even if it was created or even if there is any existence at all... Perhaps life exists in our imaginations, or even perhaps it exists in the imaginations of some other tube's imagination... anyway that's another rant...

Back to this one -

Today as this tube sees it, this tube has life to live and not a moment to spend contemplating or preparing for something other than the life it has now... there is only now... the so called 'afterlife' exists on this planet only in conversation... and only in books that were written while the authors were ALIVE!

There has never been nor will there ever be a book written by someone from the afterlife... after life comes death and death is ex-*Zackery* what it is:

Death, Worm Food, and daisy nourishment – Death.... A place where all so-called good and all so-called bad and all so-called inadequate and all so-called exemplary *tubes* finish writing their story...

Some self-inflated, self-titled, self-elevated *tubes*, who hold themselves out to be superior thinking and believing TUBES, may like to think, and have you believe, that their thoughts and ways of life are superior to yours and that there are more valid ways to spend the days you exist on this planet and that there's more to life than there really is... But when push comes to shove, the only reason they want you to believe is so they get to control some of your time on this planet to use you for their purposes and to achieve their ends.

Religion appeals to those who like to control others while pretending they're not doing what they are doing.

'Controlling others is built into the DNA of every tube that has ever lived...'

This quote is from the Book of Tubes. It's called Science and it's conducted by using test tubes.

Perhaps the existence of this tube was a test, or then again, perhaps not.

Here are the facts:

The Ten Commandments of Zackery

1. You are a *tube*, no greater or better than any other tube that lives or has lived on this planet ...
2. Tubes have what we tubes call brains... brains that are hard-wired to do whatever it takes to cause the continued existence of its host tube (the so-called body to which I am referring as a Tube).
3. Tube brains are also hard-wired to create an identity... (the proof is that every tube on the planet has an identity...) The brain is also hard-wired to do whatever it takes to cause the continued existence of itself (the identity) and the host tube (the body) on this planet.
4. Any tool, any opinion, any act, any thought, or word, be it violent or peaceful, cruel, or kind is considered fair play by tubal brains (which themselves are more tubes) in the act of causing the continued existence of their host tubes on this planet
5. You are a tube regardless of what you say is your belief. If we other tubes cut you open when you are dead or alive all we find is tubes connected to tubes connected to tubes... we tubes have been cutting open tubes for thousands of years and we have yet to find one tube that contains a belief or even an identity for that matter. Even re-birthed tubes consist of nothing but tubes.

6. You know you are a tube because you put stuff in one end and it comes out the other end.
   (The definition of a tube... Look it up in the dictionary)
7. Tube brains are very efficient at getting the existence thing handled; we engage other tubes to make it easier to continue our existences.
8. Just because a group of tubes agree that something is a particular way, doesn't make it so or make it the truth. Many tubes have agreed on many things past and present that have been proven beyond doubt by many scientific tubes to be not so, yet they continue to be in dispute and live in denial of the facts. (Take religion and the flat earth society tube gatherings, for example)
9. Pertaining to 8: Tubes are so good at existence they get bored and set off inventing new things to fill their days.
10. This tube is bored and has to go empty its bladder tube.

Are you looking forward to the next exciting adventure of the tuba?

Agendas

You saw love and experienced this love when you were a child, before society filled your heads with agendas (nothing wrong with agendas hidden or open) nothing wrong with you for having them or not having them or being aware of or not being aware of being driven by agendas you are a whole complete human being if you have agendas.

LOVE is demonstrated when you take actions that improve the quality and/or context of the life of another.

I took action - in writing this article with the agenda of improving your understanding of what it is to be a human and what the nature of love is.

I love you and my agenda here is to deliver that message.

How would you know, if you take an action today, whether that action creates a difference or makes an observable impact on anyone? You will know... your human brain will detect them as having been moved, touched, or inspired by what you did.

Did... not *thought* you did, or said or meant to do or say - if you were at all moved, touched, or inspired by what I wrote here today, demonstrate by taking an action... hit like Tony Dehn.

Consider that by declaring my agenda I have allowed the already existing love that is already present between us humans to be seen and experienced by you.

Communication is full of agendas, both hidden and explicit. Computers and cyberspace are usable as ways to avoid and to empower hidden agendas.

The grand poobah of Zackery, the Zackery same human I was yesterday, only today with one more thing written than there was yesterday. My hidden agenda... just discovered from having written this post... is to leave a legacy of thoughts and opinions for all to see, to unveil what I think, and to talk about the adventures I've experienced, both physical and mental.

Hidden agendas

For most of you I have not been at all *for* you; I have been that 'it's your job to be for you'. I don't have time for you and your stuff as I have enough of my own to worry about.

Crazy, huh?

Now that I have been told the possibility of my days being numbered, I feel the need to offer some of that time to you.

I am now for you, and here for you, if you're reading this. If you're dealing with some of the stuff that life has served you with and you're feeling that you can't do it on your own and you can pick up a phone, do so and call me...

More agenda just unfolded as I wrote that - to have you see and relate to me as the who I consider myself to be now.

I am the possibility of love and communication

I am an expression of love and confidence

I am a HUMAN who wants... Lots of friends.

Agenda for this message is to make hidden agendas clear for you, in the hope you get the message that being human is all there is... there isn't any more... regardless of who or what you or I choose to believe or follow or mimic.

Humans are very clever and the complexity and capability of the human brain is staggering, even to a human brain.

This is not evidence of a god or a creator. Actually, the fact that you need to think that is what I am writing about. What you decide as you read is the hidden agenda of which I write.

Consider the observable nature of human beings (designed, created or just evolved), in that you or I can be physically present in a situation today, whilst at the same time being driven by a background of having to get somewhere else... at work, driven by flying to get home, or to the pub... at the pub talking to a mate, whilst being driven by being (or not being) at home.

When in discussion about a subject, whilst being driven to accomplish something other than having a conversation... being in a conversation listening for an opening point, so you can have your say and being driven by the need to say it regardless of the feedback it causes.

Or one can be in the same conversation, recognizing that one's brain is simply providing that data to you to assist in the conversation - your brain isn't hard-wired to deliver that piece of advice that rattles of your tongue.

I used to (and still do) open my mouth and say stuff from my hidden agendas. I still have stuff I want to say but won't say it, (my hidden agenda is I still think you don't want to hear it) after all, I too, am human driven by a human brain...

However I have discovered that when one opens one's mouth to speak, if one observes and acknowledges (and dismisses) the hidden agenda behind the urge to speak, then what gets spoken is something that has a completely different impact upon the person to whom it is being spoken at, even when exactly the same words are used.

The tonality changes, the manner of self-importance diminishes (it doesn't disappear, you are human and they're wired with self-importance), your *occurring* to other humans listening to you alters; you become bearable...you become bearable.

Love is always present; it's part of the human condition, it doesn't have any power of its own.

Love gets blocked and stymied behind hidden agendas...

Love is allowed, it is not created or given... one allows love... one cannot choose to love another; one can allow the already-occurring love to be see-able by another by being aware of one's own hidden agendas.

Chapter 17 - Get Done what you need to Get Done

Tony

Zackery says...

How to know if you're wasting your time on this planet...

Doing is doing whether we are pretending to chase something or pretending to do nothing...

And pretending to be...

Lost is another word for 'The world's got it wrong, so I'm not playing on a round planet'.

There is nowhere to get and no one to become...

If you play, and win or lose the rat race, you're still a rat...

The real question is, are you pursuing your self-inflicted fantasy or the societal one that was spewed all over you?

How does one tell the difference? Easy...

Have you ever taken an instructed 12-month or longer course that was designed by people who have unpicked their societal web of indoctrinations?

If not, then, my friend, you are operating to the beat of someone else's drum.

And you'd be forgiven if you thought that I'm implying that you're wrong for doing so.

In a world indoctrinated and fascinated by 'There's something wrong here', there's something wrong with being told there's nothing wrong, here on Planet Round.

On Planet Round, you get the choice to walk your own path, and there is no wrong way that you take, or not take, a journey around it, even if you end up not completing your so-called journey....

Nothing wrong is a simple concept to get when you get it.

Playing someone else's drum makes the same noise whether you or they own it.

Both are valid players... regardless of the rhythm.

Neither is noble, or just, or true, or right...

Playing a drum is a thing that can be done or not done; you choose to play or not play based on your societal indoctrination, whether your society said you're a valid player that's worth listening to, or not.

Your Life is also a play opportunity.

Your life is being played by the life's that surround you and the lives of those who came before you.

And not one bit of that life was chosen by you... the 'you' who you think you are, is not who you really are.

'You' are a societal fantasy you concocted from your experiences and the rewards you received (or were denied, in your view) while playing the societal game the way your society said it should be played.

So then how does one free oneself from societal indoctrination?

Three things to do... Do!

Not read, but do!

One expresses the following three phrases...

This means you read it out loud. In other words, you speak them out loud and proud...

First,

One speaks to oneself in a mirror that...

> 'It's not wrong to have been and to continue to be indoctrinated by one's society.'

Second,

> 'It is good to feel good.'

Third,

> (this one is to be expressed with conviction in its entirety to another human with a small pause between the parts)
>
> Part 1 I am OK
>
> Part 2 You are OK
>
> Part 3 We are OK
>
> Each day say these 3 phrases to a different human being. Do this and you will become human again and joy will envelope you as it did in childhood.

Some people, let's put them in column A, seem to succeed in all fields of life. They have good relationships, great careers, read novels, don't eat sugar, call their mothers, and enjoy exercising. The others, huddled presumably less attractively in column B, drink too much, save too little, inhale carbs, buy bad presents and apply make-up to their Tube.

The desire to transition from Column B to Column A is the backbone of new years' resolutions. It is the annual mass-assumption that next year could be your year if only you made a few small changes. Unfortunately, as ambition is met with reality, many of those resolutions lie broken by the time you've finished the leftover Christmas turkey.

So we asked five experts working in the fields of fitness through to finance, how to make positive changes this New Year for a smarter, simpler, better new year.

Courageous Conversations

How to get your head in the game: Landmark is often referred to as the 'go to' for anyone looking to make a real change in their lives, be it home or work-related. Over the course of an intensive three day and one evening seminar in Euston, the international training and development company offers a lesson in self-reflection that will help you to analyse what you really want in life - and more importantly how to get it.

David Cunningham, a communication expert and seminar leader for Landmark, explains that the course works, in part, by helping participants to stop having past experiences affect their future decisions in ways that aren't productive.

> *'Things happen as we're growing up, we have experiences with money, we have experiences with success, we have experiences with failure, and then we make decisions based on those experiences - decisions like 'I'm good at this'; 'I'm not good at that'; like 'This is possible' or 'That's not possible' - and it's the decisions we make that colour and sometimes limit our choices when we are out to invent a career, or take a career step for ourselves, or take on something else important to us'.*
>
> *'First you need to be willing to think big for yourself, to be willing to say: 'Here's exactly what I want'. 'Here's exactly the kind of job I would want', says Cunningham.*
>
> *'And then distinguish or notice every reason you've got why you don't think that can happen. Then you've got a choice: you can either have what you want in life or you can have the reasons why you can't have it.'*

While it sounds simple, the reality is somewhat more challenging and the course is anything but easy. However, a bit of tough love is sometimes exactly what it takes - over two million people have taken the Landmark Forum, and the success stories continue to stack up, from CEOs to celebrities.

Here are Landmark's tips for living a more productive life:

1) Give up being right - even if you are certain that you are - and consider your viewpoint as just one possible view.
2) Be authentic - letting people in on who you really are and what you're dealing with can feel risky, but when you're straight with people and willing to be vulnerable and risk not looking good, that's the kind of conversation that has people really engage and connect.
3) Be unreasonable - practice giving up the focus on all the reasons why something can't happen. When you develop the habit of looking beyond those reasons for how you can accomplish something, you and those around you get bigger.

4) Change the way you look at problems - consider that to be alive is to have problems, you might as well make sure that your problems are big enough to be worth your time.
5) Be present - living in the moment is easier said than done. But when you can recognise the running commentary that is the thoughts and opinions that constantly pop up unbidden, and then turn down the volume on that, you are able to actually be with people, yourself, and life.

Integrity (2)

Only Integrity delivers personal power.

Where there is no integrity there is no power in the present or is there any power available to be had in the future.... When I'm not living from a created context that I have individually created... I am out of integrity and out of power to command anything to go as I say.

Integrity is honouring my word and having my word be how it goes. Having my word be how the day and the circumstances of the day go... Integrity is my honouring only a way of being which *supports how I said it would go...*

Here's an example of my Integrity list:

1. Relationships Family / friends

A: cheating on my wife
B: Lies, broken promises
C: Make wrongs

2. Finances

A: Lies on tax return
B: Not paying bills, credit cards etc
C: Not creating enough income to pay my bills and living beyond my means

3. Work / Business

A: Not making a difference as a coach
B: Only doing one coat when I quote for two
C: Doing jobs in excess of legal limitations

4. Internet

   A: Downloading pirated content
   B: copying copywritten material

5. Health

   A: Diet - Not being diligent with the diet needs of celiac
   B: Cancer ... allowing people to scam victims with mythical cures

6. Community

   A: not inviting people to forum
   B: Not following through with my commitment to launching a community affiliate book-selling business

7. Environment

   A: Washing brushes out in sinks

8. Introduction Leaders program

   A: Assignments
   B: plan of action to have my game turned out.

9. Driving

   A: Driving with road rules in mind.
   B: Vehicle Maintained to Roadworthy Certificate standard, Registration and Insurance paid up to date.

CHAPTER 18 - LIFE: FANTASY, HOPE, DESPAIR

Sally

Our family's lives have changed dramatically as do all, in a period of six years. As I write this in October 2019, I look back on the six years we as a family have ridden and continue to ride the cancer roller coaster with Tony. In the last six years, I would wait in anticipation the results of every PSA test which was at the beginning every 6 weeks once he commenced the immune treatment to see if the Zolodex was starving the cancer cells.

The PSA results showed the Zolodex still appears to be working to this day. It is not without its negative effects however. We were consulted about the side effects of this powerful drug in the beginning. The point is it's a drug which decreases the bone mineral density, which weakens your bones, not ideal for a long-term use!! We see this drug continues to have a huge impact on Tony's well-being: weight gain, muscle weakness, being out of breath after minimal exertion, and fatigue are the cost of successfully blocking the hormone which is causing the cancer to grow.

In July 2017, when we thought life was somewhat settling down, another dip in the roller coaster occurred. This is what happens when Tony has a holiday from Zolodex.

His PSA was doubling every 6 weeks. The specialist told us that the cancer had spread in the localised prostate area, and this in turn was restricting urine flow. Tony was in a huge amount of pain; he went from 2 tablets a day to 8 in a space of a week to assist urination. He was booked in for a TURPS operation.

The operation also located a mass of cancer in and below the prostate. To date, Tony has had two of these operations in a space of a year. Each time the surgeon cut away more cancer, and recovery time increased with consecutive procedures.

The next hurdle was in December 2017. We were delivered the news that as a result of a Pet scan, small cell cancer was detected. I knew that small cell cancer is a fast-growing cancer usually diagnosed with lung cancer. Early in 2018, through a biopsy, Tony found that the small cell cancer was the reason why the PSA had been doubling.

In July 2018, Paul Mainwaring referred Tony to John Flynn Hospital Oncology Unit where he was to have 8 weeks of extensive radiation (with zero guarantee that it won't grow back as soon as the treatment is finished) with gold dust injected into his prostate. This provides the radiation robot something to shoot at.

I have vivid memories of Tony coming home crying, overwhelmed with emotion at the generosity of the country Australia. The cost of the radiation was $37 K, being largely reduced to $500 out of pocket because of donations.

I found myself completely overwhelmed. I think it was a combination of caring for Tony with the TURPS operations, learning about the small cell cancer, and handling his anger and withdrawal from life in general. I found myself also wanting to run away, having time out which would allow strength to be matter of fact about sharing the news, reassuring family and friends. I knew people only meant well but I was so sick of 'how's Tony?'

I was very thankful to those who are close, forcing me to go out for breakfast, something for me, asking me how I was, just listening without judgement. I went through so many emotions, shutting myself away, finding new distractions to deflect the fact that I didn't want to deal with the impact this hideous disease. I certainly learned the importance of looking after myself. I found speaking with my GP, that my depression scale was 10. Psychologists referral, anti-depressants prescribed. I had gone down a deep hole and I knew it.

I had two psychologist appointments as well as kinesiologist's appointments which really turned the situation around. I chose to leave the script for the anti-depressants. Speaking to someone who was totally separate to the situation who provided very valuable techniques to use when I found myself not being able to breathe or sleep properly assisted immensely.

I know that it also assisted me being able to speak with close friends about what I will do when Tony passes away. Up until this point I pushed away these types of thoughts, continuing to be in denial on so many levels. I didn't want to know about it. My theory was that I would manage financially (no plan, mind you). I knew I was holding all this denial and of course Tony knew, but I had to get to being able to communicate how I felt. I have found there is no right way to feel, even writing this now in October 2019. I have raw emotions thinking of life without him. What I have learnt in the last six years is to openly communicate with Tony about the emotions I have. He is the practical one when accepting death, which assists my acceptance of the facts. Sometimes I find these conversations 'in my face', so to speak. I also find speaking about them frees up my energy which prevents my stress levels.

Tony's mission is to provide us a lifestyle to enjoy as well as providing for me and the family and to spend time with our two grandchildren. At Tony's diagnosis, were very limited in our choices. We both had life insurance policies with payout clauses for terminal illness. Tony's oncologist stated that the radiation he received would not guarantee further life expectancy beyond twelve months (which has been exceeded) and signed the paperwork allowing the claim to be approved. These funds have allowed us to invest in a property with our eldest son which we live in rent free. This also is an ongoing project to keep Tony occupied with as there are a lot of renovations to be done. Though it keeps him fulfilled, he requires reminding to take it easy when he complains that he is absolutely buggered.

We are, at the time of writing (October 2019), about to embark on a two-week cruise to celebrate Tony's 61st birthday. What a celebration, when being told at 54 that your life expectancy without treatment would be less than 12 months!

Tony

Fantasy....

My whole life has been filled with fantasies: a fantasy that I'll live to be old & grey; that I'll be rich one day; that one day I'll own a BMW; that when I have enough money I'll tour the world; that one day I'll meet the perfect woman, have the perfect life, have friends to spare and money to boot... fantasy...

OR NOT...

According to my son, I am old and grey. I've owned a Beemer; I've toured some of the world; I have the perfect wife; I have friends, I have money, I have success; I live in prosperous surroundings and I have happiness...

YET IT'S STILL NOT ENOUGH...

What is this fallacy that we need more and more and more...? I used to blame the media, now I think it's hard-wired in our beings – the need for fantasy... the need to pitch a perfect image in one's mind, an image that can't be matched and even if you came close you'd move the goal posts to keep the fantasy over reality...

GOD

If there were no humans would there be a god?

Or need for the 4000-odd gods we humans have created in our likeness?

'Why was he born so beautiful, why was he born at all?

Because he had no say in it; no say in it at all'.

My complaint is: I have no say in my life.

I have no say really in how the cancer goes or doesn't go. I have no real say in how anything goes.

Where I do have a say, it occurs as life's just too busy to give a shit about stopping me, but it will be back on the job soon.

I project that which I see...

REALITY

Perhaps it's because deep in our consciousness we know the truth about reality... reality is boring when compared to a fantasy... reality is reality and there's only so much reality we can take before we become bored with it, so we conjure up some fantasy about how it should look... how perfect my partner should be... then we run around complaining that no one measures up.

No one can measure up to a fantasy ever, not even for a moment... if they do, it's fallacy you're creating in your own mind and fallacies are in-grained with disappointment just as fantasies are, the only thing a fantasy can ever do is leave you disappointed.

Disappointment... why, then, do we crave that?

I'm loving the freedom of being free range.

Here we go - Let the drums roll and the lions roar:

Authentic:

To tell the facts or to operate how it actually is.

To state the testable, repeatable facts...

Inauthentic-

To not tell or operate with the facts

(Not how you think or feel it is,

Or *your* true story or *your* truth about it)

In-authenticity is 'holding something to be so about oneself when in fact it's not...'

Example:

'I am not good enough'... Or, 'I am beautiful',

Any way I say I am, or are, or is, is inauthentic, as it is fundamental fiction... I, or you, or some other human invented it or made it up. It wasn't true then and it certainly isn't true now...

'I wasn't good enough,' is authentic because that's past-based and in the past one has evidence to support one's case.

In the present there is no evidence to support a case for 'I am not good enough'...

And in the future, there is no future you to be admired or chastised because the future has not happened yet...

You and I are all that we ever can be right here right now, right on! Get on with the thing you say you want, regardless of your or my or society's opinion of its possibility.

Be the game!

Hope

Life is either a daring adventure or nothing.

Our preferences sometimes tend toward comfort, familiarity, safety - but in opting for those we often miss out, even to the point of giving up advancement, intimacy, adventure.

We'll have explanations as to why we hold back, telling ourselves it's easier to avoid something than it is to deal with what can be imagined, created, or committed to, and have those reasons dictate the decisions we make.

While those decisions might have the 'appearance' of freedom, they limit what's possible. When we get wrapped up in our circumstances and concerns, we can lose sight of what's possible, settle for less, and essentially adapt to things as they are.

Among the major themes to which literature repeatedly turns: love, loss, identity, ambition, none may be richer and more consuming than regret - regret about a lack of action or initiative, regret that we did or didn't express something, regret that we didn't live our lives fully.

When the possibility of power, effectiveness, and freedom arises, there's a concern we might not be able to live up to the possibility. Lack of confidence and holding back go hand in hand. Creating a breakthrough, stepping out, taking new ground requires disrupting our old conversations. There is no right place to begin, but the pull is there to move what we see or imagine as possible into action.

Real power occurs when we know we have something to say about the way things are, that we have a voice, that we have access to the state of affairs beyond just reporting on them.

When we invent ourselves by our saying, we begin an excursion into possibility.

In Helen Keller's words:

> *'Security is mostly a superstition. It does not exist in nature, nor do the children of men as a whole experience it. Avoiding danger is no safer in the long run than outright exposure. Life is either a daring adventure or nothing'.*

Choosing Vs Acceptance... Or Deciding...

One does not accept a choice!

I do not accept my choices.

It is not me doing the choosing.

In choosing, one chooses things exactly as they are in nature's reality.

From the perspective of a tree:

My decisions and opinions, my likes and dislikes, my knowledge or lack of knowledge about any matter are irrelevant in choosing, but relevant in deciding...

Choice... I Choose Death and getting dead

That does not mean I like it.

That does not mean I accept it.

It means I choose it for what it is!

Not for what I think, feel, or know about it; I do not accept it, even as I fight it to 100% of my ability.

In choosing death...

Running from it and fear of it, the grip of it, its scariness disappears.

Heartbreak ceases... And the bonus is,

All the things that death isn't become viewable...

Aliveness returns.

Like a new experience. Like the excitement of a little kid unaware of its existence.

Once again, I have the real time impact of feeling alive... I am alive and I am well and I feel great comes into my being!

Whereas before they were just words or a mantra or even worse, they were positive thinking!

May today bring you more power, freedom and self-expression for yourself and your life.

Chapter 19 - Everything and Nothing

Tony

'Hi Tony. I enjoyed reading your last post! I really appreciate your honesty and your intentions or hidden agendas. Love is the greatest and I don't know if it's just mine or every one's brain that tends to focus on the negative but it's great when peoples' hidden agenda is to inspire and show love.

Especially to the people who need it the most: The people who love u the most'.

Thanks Jon, for your comment....

This post is to detail for you the issue with the brain focusing on the negative. Firstly, focusing on the negative (as you put it) is exactly what our brains evolved to do, so you are not alone, in fact you would be alone if your brain didn't deliver you negative news...

In order to give some clarity to my above statement I offer you the following... First we must establish some facts about the brain.

Discovering I am Ape and Me

A brain function lesson.

See below lesson for conclusion -

The brain actually consists of three brains in the one skull which rides on top of a body.

The first part and largest part of the human brain is the cerebral cortex (referred to as the CC).

The second part is what's called the mid brain or the reptilian brain.

The third part is called the brain stem.

This whole package is what is commonly referred to as 'ME'. And 'ME' is where the issues with negativity begin and end. Most issues with the 'ME' stem from a lack of education about the function of the three brains and their roles.

The first part of the brain is where the identity resides - identity is the 'who you think you are and are not'... The YOU. This part also contains thinking and creative capability... This is also (contrary to popular myth) where heart, moral cognisance, sixth sense and so-called spirituality reside. This first part of the brain has no direct control over the body; it can only have an action performed by the body by sending a request to the second part of the brain.

The second part, which is known as the mid brain (MB) or the slave brain or reptilian brain, has evolved to do one thing and one thing only and that is to cause the continued existence of the 'ME'. The MB's main task is to assess and respond to danger or threats to the 'ME'... Any threat - be it real (incoming data), or imagined recycled data feed from the cerebral cortex... the CC.

The MB:

- gets its information, or incoming data, directly from the senses and the CC.
- compares the incoming data to data in its memory banks and determines the level and likelihood of danger. (So-called negative data)
- also receives and processes data of a positive nature.
- categorizes and prioritizes this data, once it has assigned a good (positive) or bad (negative) score to the incoming data.
- sends this data and its score rating to the first part of the brain

These are the things or sensations that you called negative or bad thoughts; it also processes what we call positive or good happy thoughts.

It sends this data to the CC for a deliberation from the identity that is, as a request for input or direction. The MB can and does act independently of the CC identity. If it determines the incoming data matches a known threat, or a threat that resembles a known threat, it will command the Brain Stem (BS) to act.

This third part, called the brain stem (BS) is the soldier brain; it has two jobs. Firstly, it is hard-wired to run your body, and handles all of your bodily functions automatically - like breathing, blood flow, skin replacement and so on. It doesn't think, it just acts according to its hard programming. The BS's second job is to instruct the body which is under its command to carry out the orders of the MB. Only the MB can command the BS to act. The CC can request the MB to have the BS act but the MB can refuse or deny the request.

One can, with much practice, trick the MB into doing what YOU the identity in the CC wants it to do even when it refuses. The brain deals in data via neurons firing and these neurons firing occur to us as thoughts... Better said, what we call thought is simply neurons firing inside our heads. Memories are simply clusters of neurons or patterns of neurons firing together or in sequence. When you're not remembering, those neurons of that memory are just not firing.

Conclusion.

So now to addressing so-called negative thoughts:

They are supposed to be there for YOU to deliberate on. They are just as valid as so-called positive thoughts.

Tell your MB what to do with these thoughts. If you find them invalid, tell the MB to stop sending them to you.

You do this with your voice.

Speak out loud your command, and your MB will hear the incoming data and act accordingly. The most important data that the MB responds to is the sound of your own voice.

Beware, though, of what you tell it to do, as it will carry out your command.

If the MB hears you say 'you are stupid', it will command the BS to perform stupid acts.

If it hears you tell it to be clever or be quiet it will do just that.

But note.... Don't necessarily expect, the first time that you try this, for it to work! Your MB is accustomed to one-off instances, and has learned to ignore them. If it didn't, it would be overloaded with work. And, if you have been speaking negative stuff about yourself, to yourself, for a long time and many times, your MB will have a well-worn pattern of neuronal data patterns entrenched in its data banks.

To change its response from a negative to a positive requires one more positive command, than you have given it negative commands. This means if you have told yourself 100 times that you're a bad person, it will take 101 times telling your MB that you are a worthwhile person.

Tip: never command your MB to do the opposite of a previously entrenched command. That is, never try and change from bad to good or black to white, as it will not do this task for you as this type of command is seen as a threat to the current identity of You, and it will defend the current position. To deal with this anomaly, you simply issue a different command. So bad could become worthwhile (not *good*). Angry could become something like easy, not peaceful. And you don't know how many times you have told it you're bad, you're going to have to just keep on telling it (MB) the new story until such time as the desired new behaviour manifests in the actions of your body or mind.

Tip: Do not tell your MB that you're not bad, as it will attempt to match 'not bad' within its data banks and won't be able to find a piece of data called a 'not bad', so it will assign that command to the thing which is nearest or closest to what the incoming data, which is the subject BAD, so not bad = bad (and Vice Versa not good = good)

Therefore:

1. Stop being and talking negative about your negatives, negative is natural and not wrong; in fact, it's quite right to have so-called negative thoughts.
2. Start talking to yourself about the things you do want.
3. State to yourself the who that you want you to be, and stop referring to yourself as the who that you were... and request that persons in your inner circle now refer to you as the who that YOU have chosen to be.

The who that you know yourself to be is not who you really are. The who you now know yourself to be is not fixed like a tree is fixed to the ground. You can create another way of being at any time, under any circumstances. (Circumstances to your MB are just incoming data, they just occur as real because they match the stored data in your MB). And just because the two sets of data match, doesn't make it real or make it so.

You are not a TREE... You are YOU, whole and complete and lacking nothing required to make you a whole complete human being. You are the equal of any and all human beings that have lived or are currently living or those that are yet to be born. (They will be born whole and complete just as you were).

And you've lost none of that 'whole and complete' on your journey in your life. You may have covered it up or hidden it or can't find it, or lost touch with it...

But regardless of what has happened to you (what data has entered your senses), Your wholeness is still all there.

The best story to tell oneself is:

I am whole and complete and lacking nothing.

And now something for the naysayers -

You can be rich and whole and complete and you can be poor and whole and complete. The only difference between the two is the amount of money or stuff you control, or... Better said, the amount of money that controls YOU

My Creed

I am whole and complete exactly as I am... and exactly as I am not... success is me. It is a place that I stand in. It and the who I say I am cannot be gotten to. I know that my family has my back, Always ...

Any possibility that I invent for myself and my life that I enrol others in my having gotten can be mine.

My Life is mine to create. My life cannot be found.

Each day in the morning... I stand tall and proud and say ***out loud***:

> *'I love my life and everything that is in it. Thank you, perfect universe.*
>
> *Past is Past... Present is where I am. Future is given by the perfect past that I've enjoyed.*
>
> *I am OK, you are OK and we are OK.*
>
> *I promise myself to always see others bigger than they see themselves.*
>
> *I honour my word for I know that my word differentiates me from all the tubes that inhabit this planet. I know that my word produces or reduces the sensation of the aliveness of life.*
>
> *This is my creed'.*

You have no say in what you say you want...

The You that you think you are, and your wants, were planted in your neuronal memory banks long before the you that you think you are today came into being. Once one gets to this place and accepts its truth, construction of a You designed by you can begin. And when one is at that place the world occurs as a place to dwell on, not a place to possess or attempt to own. And *Go-Getting It* disappears, because you no longer are stuck in the make-believe world of you versus *you* or *you* versus the world.

One gets to be with the order of how stuff is.

And one gets a peace that transcends the *'I want more stuff'* mindset. The desire for more life, love, happiness, success, prosperity, and money all fade from the forefront of one's mind and way of being. This reveals a life that is brimming with a respect for just being human and just being here. Happiness abounds and surrounds and envelopes with a gratitude consciousness that fills one so sufficiently that one no longer has needs or wants or dreams of wants because one has what every human searches for, from the day it is born...

Which is freedom from the dreams and desires that other humans tell us that we should do or have or be...being a human...who is at home with being human is all there is and anything else is just something to do today while I get on with being a human... Upset and despair and drama disappear from one's space and new views of what's possible appear. Not as *'have to's'*, but as realms of existence that were once unseeable by the you that you were told you were.

Zackery says...

Change is as good as a holiday and about as useful.

In every moment we make decisions,

Decisions do not get acted out.

Our choices get acted out.

Our lives have no intrinsic direction or value.

We are not boats, we don't have rudders;

Life is not a journey in which the direction can be changed.

There is nowhere to get and no one to become.

And forever is fantasy.

Death comes to everyone.

Living is the pathway to death and life is the experience one has whilst walking the path.

There is no wrong path that can be walked in life, there is no right, moral or correct path, regardless of what religion or your society says.

We didn't come from anywhere, we are nowhere, and we have nowhere to get. Life is not a journey... your life does not have to, nor should it, be any different an experience than it is for you right now.

I am ok, you are ok and we are ok.

Today's Rant!

(Inspired by a couple of posts I read today).

Death to WAR and hatred.

Life is alike, you could say, to a river that washes over each of us each day.

It brings 'things' and 'stuff' our way.

Life is what happens to us whilst we are pursuing other things.

Life has no care or concern for our cares or our concerns, about what we think about what it delivers to our doorsteps each hour, each day.

The best of life is already here and it's quite clearly screaming at us.

'I'm here! I'm here! I've been throwing life at you all of your life'.

If only we would take some time out of our pursuits of getting more out of life and pursuing and hoping for life to do our will.

If only we could let go of our concerns for how well our lives are going, we'd find the truth that our life is going...one day at a time.

Take some time today.

Time to just sit in silence and listen for life to observe life in all its magnificence.

And then to choose to appreciate what ever life has delivered to our doors without us even having to ask it to do so.

You will discover that health sickness, disease, disaster, love, sadness, complaining, grief and war and prosperity are all experiences of life, they are the rides life gives us for free.

So how's about paying life back by seeing these experiences as experiences and giving up the point of view that life didn't or hasn't delivered for you. If you've got only one complaint about something in your life, that's proof that life delivered an experience for you to complain about.

Job done, life.

Thank you, life, for adding a cancer trip to my experience and for allowing me the experience of this trip to the other side. So I get to see and play some way other than what society and I, in my pre-cancer wisdom, called normal and right for so long.

I hope you get cancer and get to deal with dying... (I bet you're glad hope doesn't work now, aren't ya?)

Perhaps then some of you would stop whingeing about what life has delivered you, and you'd get on with delivering to life what you were put here to do. You brought life to life the day you were born; you brought joy to your parents' hearts the day you were born, and have done so every day since. You can get that back by thanking your parents for getting the job done, and forgetting all the death- and dire threats you ever wished upon them. These threats, by the way, have robbed you of the joy that can be had from life.

Rekindle your love of life by getting off your story of how much wrong life and your parents did you or are doing to you. Bring life back to your life; forgive yourself for creating a viewpoint that life should go as you say, and you will find life going as you say...

Give up wishing and bringing death into yours and others' lives! Dance in and with life as if no one is watching.

Love like your heart could never be broken and if it gets broken rejoice in it having been opened once again so it can be broken again, heartbreak is a life experience. I pity those who never get to experience heartbreak for it is truly one of the most enriching experiences that I have yet had the privilege to experience.

Reach out to those you say you care about; listen with two ears and tongue in idle... And you just might get that life wants nothing to do with or to do to you and is not about you; you may then get to the position of... Life being empty and meaningless... which will get you to... You are the one who gives and brings meaning to your experiences in life... You get to say if they are labelled good or bad or inappropriate, or shouldn't have or should have... You get the say over all of the experiences that life delivers your way.

Give up all hope, give up all faith, and give away any and all thoughts of being rescued from death or from life. You may kill another but you will 'me too' within the moment you do.

Life is raining on you 24/7; you can call the rain of life refreshing or you can call it depressing. The rain of life remains, regardless of what you label it.

Even in death there is life, for without death there could not be life.

The meaning of human life is a human construct; we humans invented the word life. We gave it meaning and we get caught up in trying to control and make it go our way, this something that we made up.

I didn't say existence was meaningless.

I said the concept of life as you know it and define it is meaningless to your continued existence on this planet.

If you succeed at wiping a race of persons from this planet or from your town you will have succeeded at emptying your town or country of the empty and meaningless things that you said existed.

And you will be left with a town filled with your so-called people whose lives are in essence just as empty and meaningless as the ones you kicked out; you will have exhausted your life in the pursuit of making empty and meaningless everlasting. You will have denied yourself the love of your parents and your mends for favour from some invented construct of another human being.

Whether you enjoy what you say is a great life or a dull or boring or right and proper life... Life and the planet we inhabit derive no value from that... life is what it is and death is what it is because without it one could not have experienced life.

Neither you nor I can avoid death. We may negate it for a while but it must arrive one day for each of us in the rain of life. If your great, great, great grandparents never died you would have never got the chance to be born. There simply would not have been enough room on this planet to accommodate you. So your grands would have outlawed having children, (China has had a one child policy for decades... and they too are human just like you).

Your having a great life is meaningless to your innate hard-wired human drive for survival. The meaning of life is to get to the meaningless of life and to get present to the innate ultimate meaninglessness of the conversations that we get caught up in every day.

Getting mad is a construct

Getting even is a construct

God is a human construct

Time is a human construct

To love is human, to eat is human, to defecate is human, to get angry is human.

To kill is a construct.

To take the life of another human takes the life from you even though you may continue to walk in life and life will continue to rain on you. You will be devoid of life!

Becoming a perfect human is a human construct

You were born perfectly human and will remain perfectly human long after you're dead. No amount of prayer or worship or fasting or asking forgiveness will ever change what events or experiences life rains upon you.

Ultimately you say how your life goes.

You can go with life's flow or you can fight against life's flow... Your energies will be discharged either way...

Your experience of life will, however, be vastly different, if you fight against life with hatred, and your life will deliver you the experience of health, happiness, success, prosperity, and money along with pain and agony and grief and sorrow.

But life will deny you love.

Now get on with your life...

Get up and out and demonstrate in your actions your love for your parents and your partners and your kin and your fellow man ALL 7 BILLION OF THEM

Renounce violence and hatred as the empty and meaningless pursuits of long dead jealous men that you now know them to be... Regardless of your opinion as to their worthiness to occupy a space on this planet

Love life....

Deliver love to life

Whatever experience it brings your way...

Chapter 20 - Growths and Other Things

Tony

New paradigm for the existence of human beings...

There is only you and what you are interested in and I am not talking about you.

A you, you, you, paradigm -

In addition to the me, me, me, paradigm -

And don't mean win, win, win.

The Guru gives me a haircut

Cancer gets a haircut... (Or how to take the stench of death out of your cancer)

Cancer is a growth on or in your body just as hair is a growth in and on your body. Now I'm not saying they are the same, just that they are both growths in and on your body... Just getting clear on what relation these things are to your body...

Hair is a controllable growth.

Cancer is an uncontrolled growth.

Hair is controlled with scissors, shavers, creams, and brushes.

We haven't figured out how to control cancer yet.

We have, however, developed some tools that can kill it...

Chemo.

Lasers.

Treatments that can stall it… hormone therapy… etc etc etc…

Cancer may and does kill people.

Hair, most times, does not - although you may die from strangulation if it's long enough.

The Moral of the story:

If you be with your cancer as you be with your hair -

- Check it's ok twice a day.
- Wash it (poke it) once a day.
- Don't even notice it for 23 hours and 58 minutes of the day.

Then you will find freedom from the despair and clarity in the air that surrounds you.

With your hair, you go to the hairdressers roughly every 6 weeks for a haircut.

Treat your doctor's visits like visits to the hairdresser: a check-up to see if there's some growth or some reduction. You don't celebrate or despair regarding the growth of your hair; neither should your visit to the doctor be met with any emotional upset.

Give up being emotional: stop complaining and trying to find something wrong – or right - to lament or celebrate about your cancer.

Give up hope of being cured and you will find that automatically your despair will give up on you.

Give up the fantasy that you were supposed to live a longer life.

Who wants a life filled with fantasy, with despair and hope hanging unbearable pain and suffering in your face? Hope produces false pictures, false futures, false expectations, and false outcomes.

Get with the facts.

Cancer is a growth. Cancer doesn't cause upset.

If you're upset, then you're upset at the thought of what cancer can take from the supposed future you thought and maybe hoped would happen.

And when the fantasy walls get torn down, you're left with what human existence truly is:

Existence, survival, and relationships.

Forget survival, forget existence.

Get busy on relationships

Now, none of what I have written will enable you to stop one cancer cell from growing.

But you now have a new relationship to cancer available to you.

It may be able to kill your body...

But the memory of who you were will live strong long after you are gone in the minds and hearts of those who cross your path whilst you are still able to draw breath.

Aliveness will once again gush forth from you... just as it does from a child.

And many friends will ask... What's different about you?

Have you had a haircut?

Chapter 21 - Context is a Game Changer

Tony

Myth Busting

There's an old story that is basically true: ordinary Roman carts were constructed to match the width of ruts in the road that the war chariots had left.

The chariots were sized to accommodate the width of two large horses. Roads throughout the vast Roman Empire were all built to this specification.

When the Romans marched into Britain, roads were constructed at that width.

When the English started building tramways and railways, the width stayed the same. British labourers built railways in the Americas using the same dimensions.

Fast-forward to the space shuttle. The two large solid fuel rocket engines on the side of the launch shuttle were sent by railroad, and to be transported were designed to be the same width. A major design feature of what is arguably the world's most advanced transportation system was determined over two thousand years ago by the width of two horses.

More or less, this is an example of how knowledge can create constraints, gain momentum, and over time harden and become nearly unchangeable. Much of what we 'know' we know because someone else told us it was so. Knowledge that's handed down, inherited, is in one sense, 'everybody else's', yet we often end up living within its parameters.

We filter what we see through a somewhat distorting lens of past experience, language, and tradition. Information that has the force of history or science behind it (or just the force of habit), but doesn't fit with our existing frameworks, has a hard time being seen, heard, accepted. Add to that the notion that those frameworks have correlated frames, which further skew our view of things. What we reject and what we accept, in retrospect, often seems a bit odd.

Something keeps us in these little areas of what we already know - we call it the three-part myth of 'is, because, and I'.

- The first component of the myth is the notion of 'is', which implies that there is a 'fixed' world out there with an existence independent of us (giving us the perspective of spectator vs. player in the game). We often take for granted that things are a particular way, solid, fixed, something we have to adjust to. We become constrained and limited to what that reality allows; things are just 'the way they are'.
- 'Because' is the second component. This one can keep us caught up in a 'cause and effect' model (and thinking that's the only model). However, our actions are not always caused by something, (or an effect of something), rather they are correlated to - or in a dance with - the specific way the world shows up for us. Recognizing that takes us out of the cause-and-effect world and gives us an access to ourselves that is unavailable in the cause-and-effect loop.
- Lastly, there is the component of 'I', which refers to the who it is we consider ourselves to be (that we can get stuck with, because we mistake that for who we are). Who we consider ourselves to be is essentially arrived at by default. We put together these ways of being from a series of decisions and reactions (appropriate, perhaps, at one time), essentially built from a series of what we see (consciously or not) as failures to do or be something.

When our relationship with the world lives inside this three-part myth, we are left only with the after-the-fact realm of description, analysis, explanation - in other words, at the effect of something. Our options are only to fix, resist, change, etc., and we have no access to the full panoply available to us in being human – that is, with no power and no access to breakthroughs.

Before we can dismantle this myth, we have to recognize that it's operative. If we stop and look (at how we're being, what we're saying, etc.), we can see that we're coming from a particular place - one that gives us the set of outcomes we have.

For example, if someone tells us something's possible, and we say 'we already tried that, and it wasn't possible', our framework is likely that whatever it is 'doesn't work, and isn't going to work', and all that that implies. Seeing our operative frameworks is a bit like seeing the backs of our eyeballs. In recognizing these frameworks, though, we can shift them.

When Einstein realized, for example, that matter and energy, time and space were not separate entities, but all aspects of a whole, everything was transformed. Old knowledge took on new meaning. Breakthroughs happen not because of startling new facts, but because of a change in the overall way that the universe is seen. They require going beyond the figurable, beyond the reasonable, beyond the domain in which we 'know.'

Szymborska, a poet and Nobel laureate, said:

"Whatever possibility is, it's born from a continuous 'I don't know'.
This is why I value that little phrase so highly."

It's small, but it flies on mighty wings. It expands our lives to include the spaces within us as well as those outer expanses. If Isaac Newton had never said to himself 'I don't know', the apples in his little orchard might have dropped to the ground like hailstones and at best he would have stooped to pick them up and gobble them with gusto.

Had Madame Marie Curie never said to herself, 'I don't know', she probably would have wound up teaching chemistry at some high school.

How we hold things - our contexts, our frameworks - sets the values, limitations, and direction of our daily lives. They impose on the external world our version of reality. It can take a long time to shift our contexts, whether they're personal or those involving our relationships, our established traditions, or the culture of an enterprise-not because it takes a long time to bring about change, but because we go about it at the level of 'content.' In dealing with the content, we are extending the existing world rather than creating a new possibility in the world. We can't muck around with context with the same set of equipment we use to deal with content.

When things aren't working or we want a breakthrough, it's the context, not the content, that's the game changer.

Dealing at a contextual level puts us entirely at another level of effectiveness and creativity, and requires a different set of tools. We have something to say about the contexts we come from.

When we function at a level of context, old frames stop defining who we are. It's not that we escape them - it is rather that we escape thinking automatically, reflexively. Once we've made the distinction between how we see things and who we are, what we see becomes a function of who we are.

Nothing is more exciting than to see the world in a new way, because we don't see one new thing-we see everything in a new way. The previously unimaginable becomes possible.

* *This chapter adapted from Kevin Kelly, 'Temporary Becomes Permanent,' Kevin Kelly's Lifestream, 8-13-08, 'And from Kevin Kelly, 'Ch 0 s en, Inevitable, and Contingent,' The Technium, 7-10-09.*

CHAPTER 22 - COLLECTED THOUGHTS

Tony

Some thoughts on life... legacies for my loved ones

Free-range humaneering...

I am a Zackery... Ex-Zackery as I am... Ex-Zackery as I am not...

'A World that Works-

We can choose to be audacious enough to take responsibility for the entire human family. We can choose to make our love for the world what our lives are really about. Each of us has the opportunity, the privilege, to make a difference in creating a world that works for all of us. It will require courage, audacity and heart. It is much more radical than a revolution - it is the beginning of a transformation in the quality of life on our planet. What we create together is a relationship in which our work can show up as making a difference in people's lives. I welcome the unprecedented opportunity for us to work globally on that which concerns us all as human beings.

If not you, who?

If not now, when?

If not here, where?'

—Werner Erhard, Founder of EST Training.

Tony's Song

Taken from life-

Now that I'm gone -

Let me live on -

In your hearts and your deeds-

Taken from your life but never gone -

Think not of your needs -

But of what your fellow human needs -

The human next to you needs your love and conversation -

I am gone but your memory of me lives on.

Do justice to my last request.

Turn to a person next to you and pronounce,

'You are my friend –'

Become a friend just because you can-

Be in love with the human race -

When the otherness dissipates you will know love -

Love is actioning a difference in the quality and texture of the life of another -

To make this happen, 20 times you may have to try, and 21 times you may cry-

Put back on the shoes and go again -

When you have succeeded at this task you will understand why -

You will know what all so-called great humans know

Make the focus of your world his or hers -

And you shall be rewarded with freedom from your own fears and frustrations-

Constitute yourself as relationship –

Relationships are life -

Relationships give life and aliveness.

Be a giver of friendship -

Stay connected to the past but leave it there in the past, for that is where it belongs.

Live possibility into a future filled with Possibility unhindered by what your past says about what is or isn't possible for you and yours - Ignore your justifications for why you can't and... Just do it.

I can without the T.

Health, Happiness, Love, Success, Prosperity and Money -

These are the riches of life; these things combined bring richness to life!

They alter the experience of living for any human who takes them on at the level of constitution. (read as... The who of who you are for yourself)

To do this... read out loud the following (Please instruct the reader to instruct the audience or reader to repeat out loud the following):

I am Health... I am Happiness...I am Love... I am Prosperity... I am Success...

In life you wind up with one of two things: the results or the reason why you don't have the results. Results don't have to be explained. They just are.

Life is a game. In order to have a game, something has to be more important than something else. If what already is is more important than what isn't, the game is over.

So, life is a game in which what isn't is more important than what is. Let the good times roll.

If you could really accept that you weren't ok, you could stop proving you were ok.

If you could stop proving that you were ok, you could get that it was ok not to be ok.

If you could get that it was ok not to be ok you could get that you were ok the way you are.

You're ok, get it?

Individuals transform when there's a shift in the principle which orients their life from one of gaining satisfaction to one of expressing the satisfaction they've already got.

Only Integrity delivers personal power. Where there is integrity there is no power in the present or is there any power available to be had in the future....

When I'm not living from a created context that I have individually created...

I am out of integrity and out of power to command anything to go as I say.

Integrity is honouring my word and having my word be how it goes.

Having my word be how the day and the circumstances of the day go...

Integrity is my honouring only a way of being which *supports how I said it would go...*

To My Grandchildren - This message is for Sapphire and Jacob ...

(I request that this is read to them today and every day
of their lives until they can read it for themselves)

This is my contribution to them.

May they stand on the shoulders of giants.

Sapphire and Jacob -

I am whole and complete exactly as I am... and exactly as I am not...

Success is me...

It is a place that I stand in.

It is the who I say I am cannot be gotten to...

I know that my family has my back, Always...!

Any possibility that I invent for myself and my life that I enrol others in my having gotten can be mine...

My Life is mine to create; my life cannot be found.

Each day in the morning...

I stand tall and proud and say out loud...

'I love my life and everything that is in it...

Thank you, perfect universe...

Past is past... Present is where I am...

Future is given by the perfect past that I've enjoyed...

I am OK, You are OK, and We are OK...

I promise myself to always see others bigger than they see themselves...'

Expiration

Unit at expiry date is designed to decompose, so as not to leave a trace of manufacturer's shortcomings. Typical disposal process is by fire or burial... but worm sustenance is preferred as this dissipates the evidence of existence beyond recovery. No further contact with manufacturer is required as unit has been thoroughly tested on battlefields and love camps and has full capability of dealing with:

1. Loss of direction
2. Foul vocal emissions
3. Amnesia of origin
4. Lack of peace and joy
5. Selfish or violent behaviour
6. Depression or confusion
7. Fearfulness
8. Idolatry
9. Rebellion
10. Love
11. Joy
12. Peace
13. Patience
14. Kindness
15. Goodness
16. Faithfulness
17. Gentleness
18. Self-control

END TRANSMISSION

ABOUT THE AUTHORS

Tony

Tony was born Anthony Ernest Dehn 29th November 1958 in Melbourne, third of 8 children to mother June; first to father Gavin. His is a large, close family who stay in contact decades later. Tony recalls several locations within Victoria, from Cheltenham to Ballarat. Gavin became a career taxi-driver and supervisor; June, a dressmaker. June had a catholic upbringing, but became a Mormon while Tony was still young; Gavin followed post-retirement, together they were devout. Tony's upbringing was influenced by Mormon family values.

Tony was struck particularly by the death of his paternal grandmother when he was at a young age (he could have been seven, or eleven...); the profound impact on him was of being left, without notice or explanation.

Teenage Tony, influenced by his high school woodwork teacher, developed a life-lasting confidence in his ability to work with his hands. Tony left school at the end of 'form 5' (leaving, year 11, depending on your vintage), pursuing his part-time work at Woolworths into full-time employment. He moved into painting and decorating and, aged 20, rode his motorbike to Queensland (with a broken foot!) to work. He returned to Victoria to work as a taxi driver, age 21.

Tony believes his greatest achievements include his 3 children. He loves to traveli to Thailand to enjoy the food, lifestyle, and culture; and, of course, ocean cruising....

He has operated for most of his life either as a sole trader/ contractor, or a business owner and operator. He has enjoyed the highs of success and ridden the lows of failure. Successful or unsuccessful, Tony wakes each day to meet its challenges in the same manner: to improve.

Sally

Sally was born Sally Ann Barker 31st May 1962, at home in Houghton Regis, England; second child and only daughter to Michael and Julia Barker. Mick was a transport manager, Julie (who had worked in typing pool) a stay-at-home mum and housewife. The family included both an older and younger brother for Sally.

In June 1970 the family emigrated to Melbourne, Australia, and found accommodation in a migrant hostel. Mick found work continuing in transport management, Julie worked full-time in what would today be an administration role. The family forged a new life in a new country. There was a toll for distance and loneliness; without extended family there was always a strain on the marital relationship.

In 1973, having built and lived in a new house in Bayswater, the family sold it to bring a change of direction in ownership of a 'milk-bar', where Sally gained valuable experience in customer service and working with the public; growing confidence in her personal abilities while attending high school.

In 1977 her parents separated and consequently sold the business.

For a short time, Sally lived with her father and younger brother, settling into a housekeeper/ daughter role while still at school. Sally left high school at the end of 'form 4' (year 10) to continue study at a secretarial college.

Sally had left home by the time Mick met his next wife, and was working for a florist. She later moved into the taxi industry as a radio operator....

Sally thrives on a challenge and has always responded positively to what is thrown in front of her. She enjoys travelling and its memories, the company of friends, and, in later years, watching AFL.

Together

Tony and Sally met working for a taxi-company; he was driving taxis and she was a radio operator. It was the early 1980s – he was 24, she might have been 21....

Their life together grew very quickly. They were married in October 1985. With the strong encouragement and support of Tony's father Gavin, they moved into the business of owning and operating a regional taxi company. The flair for growth never far away, the business developed and flourished. At one stage their business boasted 9 vehicles across 3 towns - they operated it for 12 years before moving on.

During this time, or thereabouts, they also involved themselves in direct selling in different ways, gaining exposure to different business models and business practises. They worked very hard at whatever enterprise was on the go. Post-taxis, Tony moved into independent business coaching, using his experience as a business owner, and the influence and training of Brad Sugars, to help develop and grow diverse businesses.

Their family was also growing. A ten-year participation in Melbourne's IVF program assisted in delivering three healthy children, including twins, which made life very busy. Sally and Tony now have grandchildren who they both adore. They have always whole-heartedly immersed themselves in life's experiences, and continue to support their children and grandchildren in their lives.

While Gavin and June devoted themselves to being Mormons, and Sally had supported Julie into becoming an enthusiastic born-again apostolic Christian, Tony and Sally each individually participated in the Landmark Forum in 2001. Together they had developed with the training delivered through Landmark Education: clear-thinking and logic separated from the clutter inherent in being human.

At the age of 46, after battling odd fatigue and mysterious symptoms including blotchiness, bloating and various gastric complaints, Tony was eventually diagnosed with coeliac disease. Working in his business coaching business, encountering societal ignorance of his condition, and for the better health of all concerned, the family re-located to the warmer climes of Queensland's Gold Coast.

New vocations ensued. Tony used his practical skills in business as a handyman, while still actively pursuing other business interests through coaching as well as exercising his entrepreneurial bent. Sally worked in vocational training and placement, including through the trauma of an employer liquidating, until being herself struck with a physical limitation resulting in many surgeries and recoveries. Their children grew up. Sally and Tony still live on the Gold Coast.

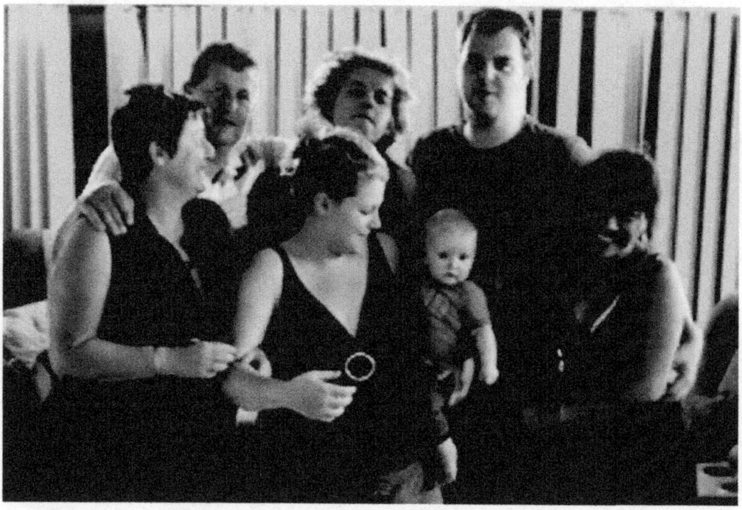